Table Of Contents

50 EASY DIABETIC DESSERT RECIPES
by STELLA WATERS

Do you miss being able to eat something sweet every once and awhile?

A diabetes diagnoses usually means that you can no longer eat sweets or other sugary desserts ever again. This book is filled with all sorts of cakes, brownies and other delicious desserts that will have you looking forward to staying on your diabetic diet.

This book contains everything that you have a missed eating, now back with diabetic safe recipes, so you can enjoy them just like you used too. And best of all, your family can too; these sweet and savory desserts are so good that most people can't tell the difference. Best of all, no matter the celebration, holiday or family event, you will be able to bring a delicious, diabetic safe dessert.

If you are tired of eating the same old diabetic diets, then you need this book. Filled with tons of family favorite recipes which have been reworked to taste great and be diabetic safe. Unlike other books, these recipes are all about taste, if it does not taste great then it is not in the book.

The reason for this is that great recipes are meant to be shared with those closest to you, whether they are diabetic or not. That way, you and your family can eat cake and share cookies together, just like you used to.

What's in this book?

- ➢ Muffins
- ➢ Cakes
- ➢ Cookies
- ➢ Sweet Fat-Bombs
- ➢ Desserts
- ➢ Snacks and Treats
- ➢ Diabetic Fruity Desserts

■ **Diabetic Safe Pies:**
Everything from Apple Pie to Lemon Cream Pie all made so you can eat it without worries.

■ **Diabetic Safe Cakes and Brownies:**
From Carrot Cakes to Chocolate Brownies, these recipes are so good that diabetics and non-diabetics both can enjoy it.

■ **Diabetic Safe Cookies:**
From Banana Cookies to Gingersnap's, this book has enough cookie recipes to keep you and your family happy for years.

Thanks for choosing this book, make sure to **leave a short review** on Amazon if you enjoy it. I'd really love to hear your thoughts

Enjoy! 😊

Stella Waters.

EASY

DIABETIC

DESSERT

RECIPES

CHOCO FAT BOMBS

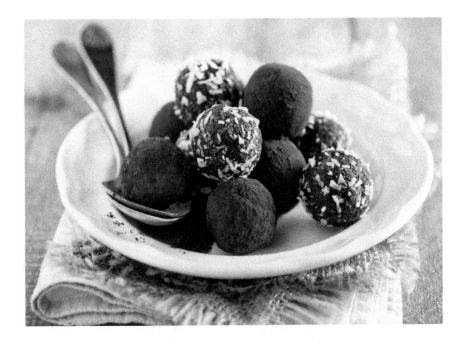

Choco Fat Bombs is a great recipe to increase your fat intake and help satisfy your chocolate cravings. If you need a savory diabetic dessert recipe, this Fat Bomb is the right recipe to have.

I highly recommend trying this dessert. It's packed with awesome flavor and it's incredibly easy. To make this recipe, all you need is your fridge or freezer, a bowl, and a tray with parchment paper.

INGREDIENTS

- 2 tablespoons of heavy cream
- 1 teaspoon of vanilla extract
- 2 tablespoons of Stevia
- 1/4 cup of unsweetened cocoa powder
- 5 tablespoons of natural chunky peanut butter
- 6 tablespoons of hemp seeds (shelled)
- 1/2 cup of unrefined coconut oil

PREPARATIONS

- Mix peanut butter, cocoa powder, and hemp seeds in a large bowl.
- Add room temperature coconut oil and mix till it becomes a paste.
- Add vanilla, cream, and stevia. Mix until it becomes a paste again.
- Roll into balls. When rolling, you should make up to 12 balls in total.
- Put in the fridge, if the paste is too thin to roll, for about 30 minutes before rolling.
- Roll in shredded coconut.
- Place balls on parchment paper on a baking tray.
- Put in the fridge for at least 30 minutes before serving.
- Serve and enjoy.
- Store the leftover in the fridge.

PREP TIME : 15 mins
FREEZE TIME : 10 mins
TOTAL TIME : 25 mins
YIELD : 12 balls

LOW-CARB CHEESECAKE

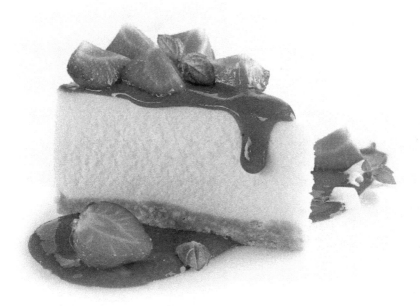

This healthy Low Carb Cheesecake is a simple and delicious recipe to make. This cheesecake recipe is the right answer to your cravings. It helps satisfy your cheesecake cravings without blowing a whole week's calorie budget.

For a cake with almost no fat, calories, or carbs, it tastes absolutely amazing. You'll always get high praise when you serve it to your health-conscious families and friends.

They will love it. I promise!

- 1 tablespoon of stevia
- 1 teaspoon of vanilla extract
- 1 serving of sugar-free Strawberry Jell-O
- 8.5 ounces of low-fat cottage cheese
- 2 egg whites
- 1 scoop vanilla protein powder
- Water

- Preheat the oven to 325 degrees F.
- Prepare the Jell-O according to the package directions.
- Place in the freezer.
- Blend egg whites and cottage cheese until the consistency is smooth.
- In a bowl, pour the blended mixture, and whisk it together with the stevia, protein powder, and vanilla extract.
- In a small nonstick pan, transfer the batter. Bake for about 25 minutes.
- Turn off the oven.
- Leave the cake in the oven while it cools down.
- Remove the cheesecake from the oven once it has cooled.
- Pour it over the cheesecake when the Jell-O is almost set (you should be able to stir it).
- Let the cake set in the fridge before serving, for about 10 hours minimum.
- Serve and enjoy.

PREP TIME : 10 mins
COOK TIME : 50 mins
TOTAL TIME : 1 hour
YIELD : 2 servings

PROTEIN BUTTER COOKIES

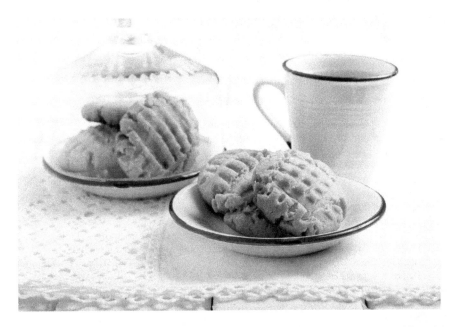

I believe a healthy diabetic diet should absolutely include dessert. So, if you're looking for the best cookies to enjoy, these Peanut Butter Cookies are a healthy way to satisfy your cookie craving after having your breakfast or lunch meal.

They taste good and they come together in a bowl with just five ingredients for a super treat.

- 2/3 cup of erythritol
- 1/2 teaspoon of baking soda
- 1 cup of smooth peanut butter (no added sugar)
- 1 large egg
- 1/2 teaspoon of vanilla essence

PREPARATIONS

- Preheat oven to 350 degrees F.
- Use baking paper to line a cookie tray and set it aside.
- Add the erythritol into a blender or nutribullet.
- Blend until powdered and set it aside. You can skip this step if you'll be using a confectioner's low-carb sweetener.
- In a medium mixing bowl, add all of the ingredients and mix until a glossy smooth dough forms.
- Roll about 2 tablespoons of dough between your palms to form a ball.
- Then place on the prepared cookie tray.
- Repeat until all dough has been used. You should end up with 12 to 15 cookies.
- Flatten the cookies using a fork, creating a crisscross pattern across the top.
- Bake for about 12 to 15 minutes.
- Remove from the oven.
- Allow to cool on the baking tray, for about 25 minutes.
- Then transfer into a cooling rack for another 15 minutes.
- Serve and enjoy.

PREP TIME : 5 mins
COOK TIME : 15 mins
FREEZE TIME : 40 mins
TOTAL TIME : 1 hour
YIELD : 12 servings

RASPBERRY MUFFINS WITH PUMPKIN

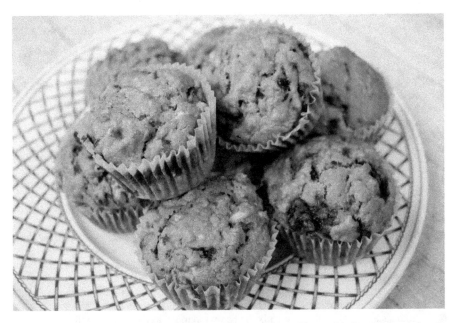

Nobody will believe that this particular Raspberry Muffins with Pumpkin recipe is actually low-fat, low-carb, sugar-free, and diabetic friendly. They won't believe it until you tell them.

They are very simple to put together, and also, they will become a family favorite for either breakfast, lunch boxes, or snacks. This dessert recipe can be shared at parties and you would have fun watching people eating them and praising you.

- 1 cup of pumpkin puree - canned
- 1/2 cup of coconut flour
- 3/4 cup of blanched almond flour
- 1/2 cup of Stevia
- 1/4 teaspoon of salt
- 4 (1/2 cup) egg whites
- 4 egg yolks
- 1/2 cup of coconut oil (melted)
- 1 1/2 teaspoon of vanilla extract
- 1 1/2 cup of frozen raspberries
- 10 drops of liquid stevia
- 3 tablespoons of arrowroot starch or tapioca
- 1 tablespoon of baking powder
- 1 tablespoon of cinnamon
- Pinch nutmeg

PREPARATIONS

- Preheat your oven to 350 degrees F.
- Use muffin papers to line 12 muffin cups.
- Stir together the almond flour, coconut flour, tapioca starch, stevia, cinnamon, baking powder, sea salt, and nutmeg in a large bowl until it is all mixed well.
- Stir in the pumpkin puree, stevia drops, coconut oil, vanilla and egg yolks (keep the egg whites separate for the next step) until completely incorporated.
- Beat the egg whites in a separate bowl until stiff white peaks form.
- Fold the frozen raspberries and egg whites into the muffin batter.
- At this stage, make sure to not mix the batter too much as the muffins will become denser if you do.
- Fold the egg whites and raspberries gently into the batter, using spatula or a spoon.
- Spoon the muffin batter into the muffin papers.
- Smooth out the tops.
- The batter should just be at the top of the muffin papers.
- Keep the muffin papers fuller to compensate as the muffins don't rise very high.
- Bake muffins for about 25 minutes.
- On the top of the muffins, it will be a light golden. Also, the toothpick should come out clean when inserted.
- Allow it to cool for about 5 minutes in the muffin tray before placing the muffins on a cooling rack to cool completely.
- Serve and enjoy.

PREP TIME : 10 mins
COOK TIME : 25 mins
COOL TIME : 20 mins
TOTAL TIME : 1 hour
YIELD : 12 muffins

STRAWBERRY POPSICLES WITH LEMON

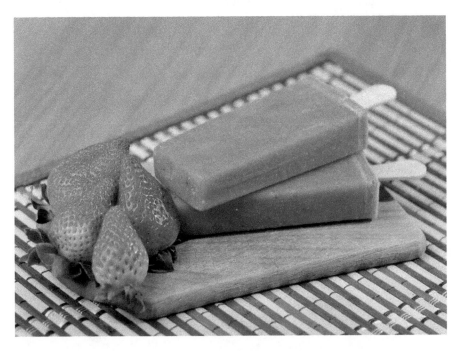

These healthy Strawberry Popsicles with Lemon have all the delicious flavors of a summer treat with zero sugar added. And with just five ingredients, your dessert will be ready to consume.

What makes this recipe unique are the old-fashioned oats and low-fat cottage cheese. Although, strawberries, stevia extract, and lemon juice are ingredients you would expect. I hope you love it, seriously.

They are a treat that anyone can feel good about eating, especially for people with diabetes like me.

- 4 ounces of low-fat cottage cheese
- 1 and half pound of strawberries
- 1/4 cup of old-fashioned oats
- 4 ounces of lemon juice, (about 4 lemons)
- 5 drops of liquid Stevia

PREPARATIONS

- In a high powdered food processor or blender, pulse the oats until they turn into powder.
- Add the cottage cheese, strawberries, stevia and lemon juice.
- Then pulse until smooth.
- Stop the blender if necessary.
- Use a spatula to push the ingredients down.
- Do not add any liquid.
- Pour the mixture into your 6 Popsicle molds.
- Freeze for at least 3 hours, until solid.
- Serve and enjoy.

PREP TIME : 5 mins
FREEZE TIME : 3 hours
TOTAL TIME : 3 hours 5 mins
YIELD : 6 servings

KETO CHOCO FUDGE

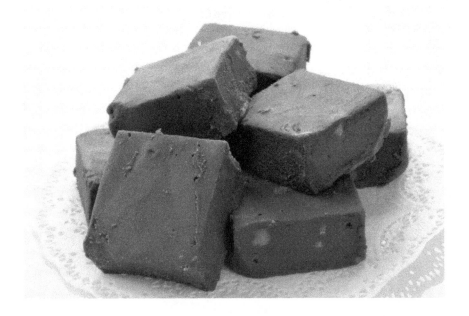

This Keto Choco Fudge is so simple and it just happens to be keto, vegan, low carb, and diabetic-friendly.

This recipe is so dangerously easy, it takes just three simple ingredients and five minutes to be ready to eat. You just have to let it sit in the fridge for some hours. You know what I mean, right? You'll love it that way.

The result is creamy, smooth, and rich. I hope you love it.

Enjoy.

INGREDIENTS

- 10 ounces of bittersweet chocolate chips
- 1 1/2 cups of coconut butter
- 1 (13.66 FL ounces) can of full-fat coconut milk
- Optional: coarse or flaked sea salt for topping

PREPARATIONS

- Use foil or wax paper to line an 8 by 8-inch baking pan.
- Melt the coconut butter over low heat in a small saucepan.
- Stir in the chocolate chips and coconut milk.
- Cook over low heat, until the chocolate chips are melted.
- Stir frequently when cooking.
- Pour the mixture in a pan.
- Optional: Sprinkle coarse or flaked sea salt over the top.
- Place in the refrigerator for about 2 hours, until set.
- Slice and enjoy.

PREP TIME : 5 mins
CHILL TIME : 2 hours
TOTAL TIME : 2 hours 5 mins
YIELD : 40 squares

BANANA COOKIES

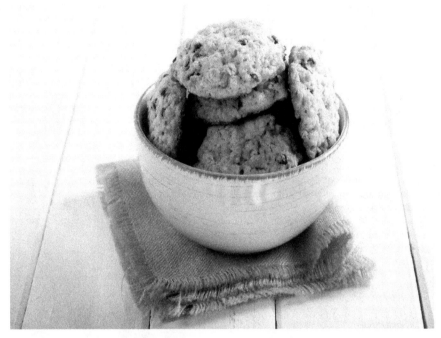

You don't need to change anything whatsoever in this recipe at all. The cookies tasted a bit like banana bread because of the cinnamon. This recipe will definitely rival yours. It's a great recipe you need to try today.

They are quite filling and make a great snack in the middle of the day. Do you know what I love about this recipe? My dear, you can get addicted to them. Lol.

I hope you love it.

INGREDIENTS

- 1 cup of raisins
- 1/3 cup of plain yogurt
- 3 very ripe bananas
- 2 cups of rolled oats
- 1 teaspoon of ground cinnamon

PREPARATIONS

- Preheat the oven to 350 degrees F.
- Use parchment paper to line cookie sheets.
- In a large bowl, mash bananas.
- Add raisins, yogurt, oats and cinnamon.
- Mix well.
- Allow it to sit for 15 minutes.
- Drop spoonful's of dough 2 inches apart onto the prepared cookie sheets.
- Bake in the preheated oven for about 20 minutes, until browned lightly.
- Serve and enjoy.

PREP TIME : 10 mins
CHILL TIME : 20 mins
ADDITIONAL TIME : 15 mins
TOTAL TIME : 45 mins
YIELD : 12 cookies

STRAWBERRY GRANITA

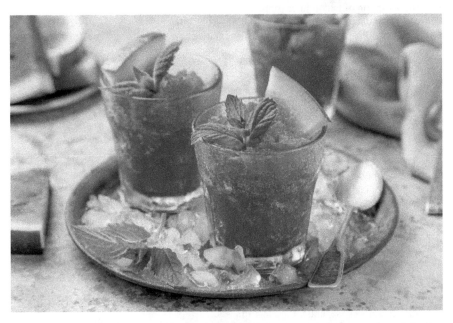

You can make this dessert recipe and serve anytime. But it is best enjoyed during the summer periods. It's extremely delicious and creamy, but heavy. This recipe is a great way to use an abundance of strawberries from your garden patch. Please make sure you eat this as a summer refresher :)

It's very simple and make sure to leave enough time for the freezing and stirring. You can make it in the morning and it will be ready to consume in the summer evenings.

Please make sure you don't omit the balsamic vinegar. This is because it adds brightness to the dish.

INGREDIENTS

- 1 cup of water
- 1/2 teaspoon of lemon juice (optional)
- 1/4 teaspoon of balsamic vinegar (optional)
- 2 pounds of ripe strawberries, halved and hulled
- 1/3 cup of white sugar, or to taste
- 1 tiny pinch of salt

PREPARATIONS

- Use cold water to rinse the strawberries.
- Transfer the berries into a blender.
- Add water, sugar, lemon juice, salt, and balsamic vinegar.
- To get the mixture moving, you need to pulse several times.
- Blend for about 1 minute, until smooth.
- Pour into a large baking dish (in the dish, the puree should be about 3/8 inch deep).
- In the freezer, place dish uncovered until mixture barely starts to freeze for about 45 minutes, around the edges.
- Mixture will still be slushy in the center.
- Stir the crystals from the edge of the granita mixture lightly into the center and mix thoroughly using a fork.
- Close freezer and chill for about 30 to 40 minutes, until granita is nearly frozen.
- Lightly mix with a fork before scraping the crystals loose.
- Repeat with freezing and stirring with fork until the granita is light, looks fluffy and dry, crystals are separate, for 3 to 4 times.
- Portion the granita into small serving bowls.
- Serve and enjoy.

PREP TIME : 10 mins
FREEZING TIME : 2 hours 10 mins
TOTAL TIME : 2 hours 25 mins
YIELD : 8 servings

BAKED APPLES

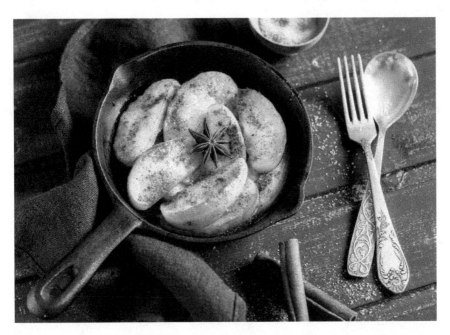

This easy Baked Apple recipe makes a great snack and/or dessert. You can use whatever fruit-flavored diet soda that catches your fancy.

This recipe is great with the diet orange. You can use diet Crush. You would smell the orange by the time you open the oven. Whipping with cream or strawberry yogurt on top is also a great way to enjoy this recipe.

INGREDIENTS

- 2 cups of sugar-free diet orange-flavored carbonated beverage
- 6 small apples, halved and cored

PREPARATIONS

- Preheat an oven to 350 degrees F.
- Arrange the apples into a baking dish with the cut sides facing down.
- Over the apples, pour the orange beverage.
- Bake in the preheated oven for about 1 hour, or until the apples are tender.
- Serve and enjoy.

PREP TIME : 5 mins
COOK TIME : 1 hour
TOTAL TIME : 1 hour 5 mins
YIELD : 6 servings

BANANA CHIA PUDDING

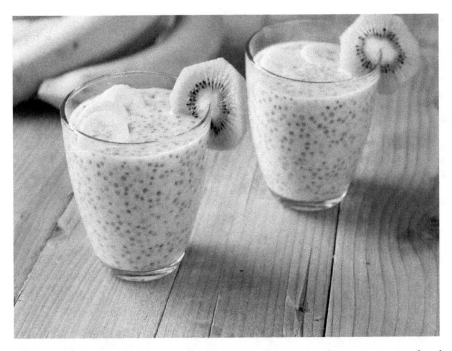

Banana Chia Pudding is the kind of diabetic dessert that is so easy to make, is delicious, and all-around awesome. You can use vanilla soy milk instead and making this recipe on a fairly regular basis would be great.

You'll never regret it. It's a fantastic snack with so many health benefits. It's awesome and delish.

Enjoy.

INGREDIENTS

- 3 tablespoons of honey
- 1 teaspoon of vanilla extract
- 1/8 teaspoon of sea salt
- 1 and 1/2 cups of vanilla-flavored flax milk
- 1 large banana, cut in chunks
- 7 tablespoons of Chai seeds

PREPARATIONS

- In the blender, put these in respective order: milk, banana, chia seeds, honey, vanilla extract, and sea salt.
- Blend together until smooth.
- Pour mixture into a bowl.
- Refrigerate for at least 2 hours, until thickened.
- Spoon mixture into small bowls to serve.
- Serve and enjoy.

PREP TIME : 10 mins
COOK TIME : 2 hours
TOTAL TIME : 2 hours 10 mins
YIELD : 6 servings

MEXICAN MANGO

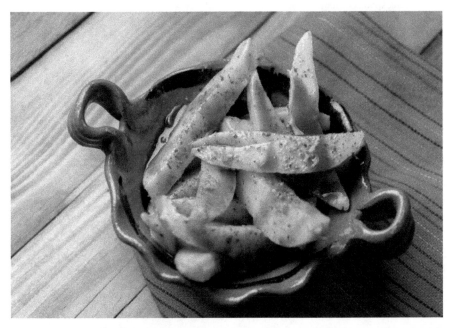

If you want to enjoy this Mexican Mango, you can make it in the morning, cool it and put it in the refrigerator. Then at dinner, heat it for a couple of seconds in the microwave. In fact, you can just double the recipe. You'll definitely add it to your favorites.

You can serve with coconut shrimp and steak. So nice and delicious.

- 1 pinch of salt
- 3 tablespoons of lemon juice
- 1/4 cup of water
- 1 tablespoon of chili powder
- 1 mango - seeded, peeled, and sliced

PREPARATIONS

- In a small saucepan, bring water to a boil.
- Stir in salt, chili powder, and lemon juice until hot and smooth.
- Add sliced mango and toss to coat.
- Allow it to soak up the chili sauce for some minutes before serving.
- Serve and enjoy.

PREP TIME : 5 mins
COOK TIME : 10 mins
TOTAL TIME : 15 mins
YIELD : 2 servings

BANANA ICE CREAM

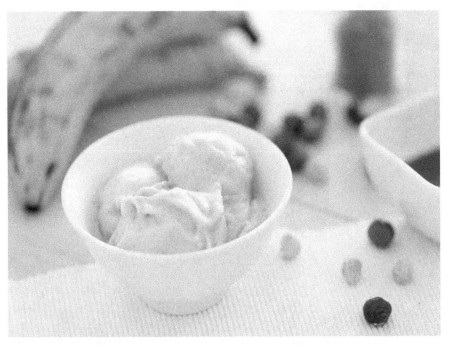

Please do not throw your banana away when they are overripe. All you need to do is peel them, wrap them in plastic wrap, and freeze them. Only two ingredients is all you need to make this family pleaser.

Enjoy.

INGREDIENTS

- 1/2 cup of skim milk
- 2 chopped and peeled bananas, frozen

PREPARATIONS

- Combine 1/4 cup of skim milk and frozen bananas in a blender.
- Blend for about 30 seconds.
- Add remaining 1/4 cup of milk.
- Blend for about 30 seconds on high speed until smooth.
- Serve and enjoy.

PREP TIME : 5 mins
COOK TIME : 0 mins
TOTAL TIME : 5 mins
YIELD : 2 servings

APPLE PIE

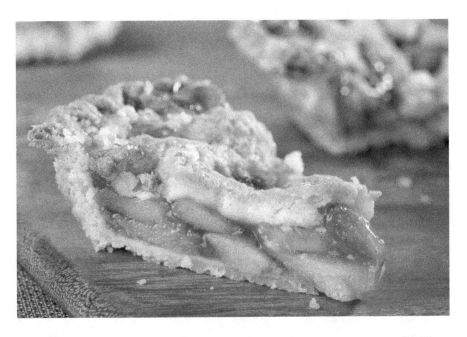

For this recipe, using apple juice is a great idea. When you use sugar substitutes, the pie will seem dry - that would help solve that problem.

Make this recipe for your family's thanksgiving feast. No one in the family group will even know this is a diabetic Apple Pie.

You can stick to your apple juice flavor. It'll give the pie a really nice added flavor. What I love about this recipe is that it will be great the next day.

INGREDIENTS

- 1/3 cup of thawed apple juice concentrate
- Pastry for double-crust pie (9 inches)
- 8 cups of thinly sliced peeled tart apples
- 1 tablespoon of butter
- Sugar substitute equivalent to 8 teaspoons of sugar
- 2 teaspoons of cornstarch
- 1 teaspoon of ground cinnamon

PREPARATIONS

- Combine the apple juice, sugar, cornstarch, and cinnamon together.
- Line a pie plate with a bottom crust; add apples.
- Over the apples, pour juice mixture and dot with butter.
- Roll out the rest of the pastry to the fit top of pie.
- Cut slits or an apple shape in top.
- Place over filling; flute and seal edges.
- Bake at 375 degrees for about 35 minutes.
- Increase heat to 400 degrees.
- Bake until apples are tender for about 15 to 20 minutes.
- Serve and enjoy.

PREP TIME : 15 mins
BAKE TIME : 50 mins
TOTAL TIME : 1 hour 5 mins
YIELD : 8 servings

GRILLED PEACHES

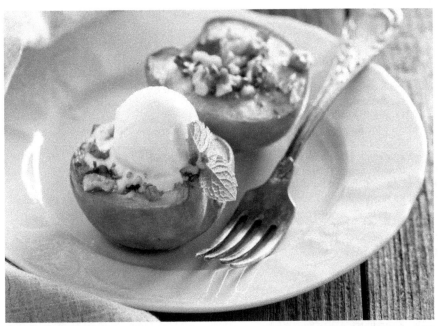

Grilled peaches are the kind of magic that happens in a hot grill's twilight, and it's the best pairing for the cold wine and ice cream destined for dessert.

The truth about these grilled peaches is that they are surprisingly simple, and they just require olive oil and fresh peaches to prepare on a cooling grill.

The finished peaches should not be falling apart with distinct grill marks and it should be more tender. Actually, most of the peach skin will be slipping away and you just need to pull these off using your tongs before serving if you feel like it. Enjoy.

- 6 peaches (freestone)
- Olive oil

Preparing the grill:
- Light a gas grill to medium heat.
- Grill the peaches after everything else has been grilled. That is if you'll be cooking over charcoal.

Making the grilled peaches:
- Halve the pit of peaches by running a sharp knife along each of the peach's seam to halve them.
- Remove the pit and use olive oil to brush each cut side.
- Place the peaches cut side down on the grill.
- Cook undisturbed for about 4 to 5 minutes, until grill marks appear.
- Flip the peaches, then grill for about 4 to 5 minutes more, until the peaches are soft and skins are charred.
- Remove from the grill.
- Serve the grilled peaches with butter or vanilla ice cream.
- Enjoy.

PREP TIME : 5 mins
COOK TIME : 10 mins
TOTAL TIME : 15 mins
YIELD : 8 servings

PEANUT BUTTER SWIRL BROWNIES

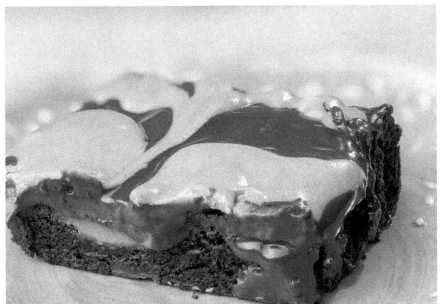

This diabetic-friendly brownie recipe uses the classic combination of peanut butter and chocolate to make a delicious dessert you will want to make again and again.

It's not too cakey and not too fudgy. But sincerely, you would love it.

Enjoy!

INGREDIENTS

- 1 teaspoon of vanilla
- 1 1/4 cups of whole-wheat pastry flour, divided
- 1 teaspoon of baking powder
- 1/4 cup of creamy peanut butter
- 1/2 cup of unsweetened cocoa powder
- Nonstick cooking spray
- 1/4 cup of butter
- 3/4 cup of granulated sugar
- 1/3 cup of cold water
- 3/4 cup of refrigerated or frozen egg product, thawed, or 3 eggs (lightly beaten)
- 1/4 cup of canola oil
- 1/4 cup of miniature semisweet chocolate pieces

PREPARATIONS

- Preheat the oven to 350 degrees F.
- Use foil to line a 9x9x2 inch baking pan, extend foil up over the edges of the pan.
- Use nonstick spray to lightly coat foil and set it aside.
- Melt butter in a medium saucepan over low heat.
- Remove from heat.
- Whisk in the water and sugar.
- Whisk in oil, egg, and vanilla until combined.
- Stir in the baking powder and 1 cup of the flour until combined.
- In a small bowl, place the peanut butter; gradually whisk in 1/2 cup of the batter until smooth and set it aside.
- Combine the cocoa powder and the rest 1/4 cup of flour in a separate bowl.
- Stir into the plain batter.
- Stir in chocolate pieces and pour the chocolate batter into the prepared pan.
- In small mounds, drop peanut butter batter over chocolate batter in pan.
- Swirl batter together using a thin metal spatula.
- Bake until a toothpick inserted in the center comes out clean and the top springs back when lightly touched, for about 20 to 25 minutes.
- Cool completely in a pan over a wire rack.
- Cut into bars.
- Serve and enjoy.

PREP TIME : 15 mins
COOK TIME : 0 mins
TOTAL TIME : 40 mins
YIELD : 20 servings

ALMOND QUINOA BLONDIES

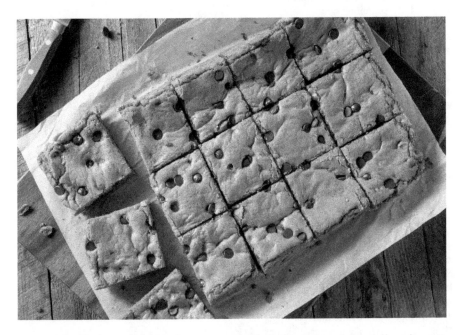

More than likely, people won't even notice that these chocolaty, delicately nutty blondies are diabetic and gluten-free.

They use quinoa flour which you can find in natural food stores and well-stocked supermarkets, in the place of all-purpose flour. If you want to make your quinoa flour, you can grind raw quinoa into a powder using a clean coffee grinder.

You can use almond extract instead of vanilla. It will still add a lovely flavor to this dessert. Enjoy.

INGREDIENTS

- 1 teaspoon of vanilla extract
- 3/4 cup of quinoa flour
- 1 teaspoon of baking powder
- 1/4 teaspoon of salt
- 1/4 cup of unsalted butter, softened
- 3/4 cup of crunchy or smooth natural almond butter
- 2 large eggs
- 3/4 cup of packed light brown sugar
- 1 cup of semisweet chocolate chips

PREPARATIONS

- Preheat oven to 350 degrees F.
- Use parchment paper or foil to line an 8-inch square baking pan.
- Allow it to overhang opposite ends slightly.
- Use cooking spray to coat.
- Beat almond butter and butter in a bowl until creamy using an electric mixer.
- Beat in brown sugar, eggs and vanilla.
- Whisk baking powder, quinoa flour, and salt in a small bowl.
- Mix the flour mixture into the wet ingredients until just combined.
- Stir in chocolate chips.
- Evenly spread the butter into the prepared pan.
- Bake for about 25 to 35 minutes or until a toothpick inserted into the center comes out with just some little moist crumbs.
- Do not overbake it.
- Let it cool in the pan for about 45 minutes.
- Lift the whole pan out using the parchment or foil and transfer to a cutting board.
- Cut into squares and serve and enjoy.

PREP TIME : 15 mins
COOL TIME : 1 hour 20 mins
TOTAL TIME : 1 hour 35 mins
YIELD : 24 servings

FRUIT YOGURT POPSICLES

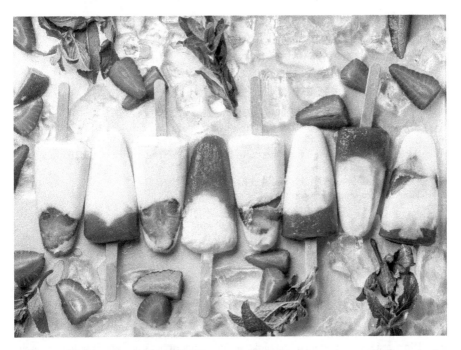

These popsicles have more strawberry than the yogurt. You can increase the amount of yogurt to 1 and a half cups if you would like closer to equal parts of strawberry and yogurt. Balancing the berries and yogurt will make you love this recipe.

These are not only great for snacks, but for dessert as well. I hope you enjoy it.

For the simple syrup:
- 1/2 cup of water
- 1/2 cup of granulated sugar

For the Popsicles:
- 1 tablespoon of lemon juice
- 1 cup of plain or vanilla yogurt
- 1 pound (4 cups) of strawberries, halved and hulled

PREPARATIONS

- In a saucepan, stir the water and sugar together over medium heat.
- Bring to a boil and stir till the sugar dissolves.
- Chill until cold.
- Puree the strawberries, 3 tablespoons of the syrup and lemon juice in a food processor or blender until smooth.
- Taste and add more syrup if you feel like.
- Transfer into your measuring bowl or cup.
- Whisk the yogurt to smooth out the lumps in a bowl.
- Fill the molds by alternating 1 tablespoon of yogurt and 1 tablespoon of fruit.
- Continue alternating berries and yogurt until the molds are filled to 1/4-inch from the top.
- Poke deep into popsicle molds and swirl yogurt with fruit together using a chopstick or skewer.
- Freeze for an hour.
- Remove the mold from the freezer and insert the popsicle sticks inside, leaving about 2-inch of each stick above the mold.
- Return to the freezer until frozen, for another 3 hours.
- Dip the sides and bottom of the mold in a container of hot water and hold long enough to thaw the popsicles so they release from the mold.
- Serve and transfer into the store in the freezer.
- Enjoy.

PREP TIME : 10 mins
FREEZING TIME : 5 hours
TOTAL TIME : 5 hours 10 mins
YIELD : 10 popsicles

BAKED CINNAMON STUFFED IN APPLES

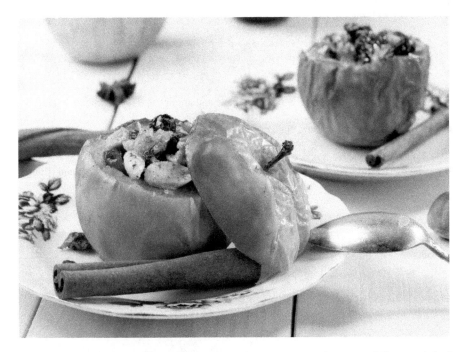

Yummy apples with oatmeal filling are a great way to enjoy your fall tree-picked apples.

Let me tell you something; this recipe is so delicious and perfect. A scoop of vanilla ice cream sends it over the top. You won't want to change this recipe because they are tender, juicy and can be ready within 30 minutes.

Your whole house will smell wonderful by the time you place the apples in the oven.

INGREDIENTS

- 4 apples
- 1 teaspoon of ground cinnamon
- 1/4 cup of butter
- 1 cup of rolled oats
- 1/4 cup of brown sugar

PREPARATIONS

- Preheat the oven to 350 degrees F.
- Core each of the apple.
- Make a large well in the center of each apple and arrange them on a rimmed baking sheet.
- Mix brown sugar, oats, and cinnamon together in a bowl.
- Cut in butter until evenly combined.
- Spoon 1/4 of the oat mixture into each apple.
- Bake in the preheated oven for about 30 minutes, or until apples are tender and filling is bubbling.
- Serve and enjoy.

PREP TIME : 15 mins
COOK TIME : 40 mins
TOTAL TIME : 45 mins
YIELD : 4 servings

DARK CHOCO ALMOND BARK

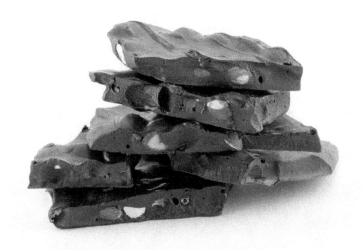

Dark Choco Almond Bark is a great treat for diabetics.

Adding sea salt to this treat would be great too. The combination of Dark Choco Almond Bark with sea salt will definitely satisfy your craving. And you would want to double your recipe because it doesn't last long.

Well, I hope you enjoy it too.

INGREDIENTS

- 1/8 teaspoon of sea salt
- 1/2 teaspoon of vanilla extract
- 1/4 cup of almonds chopped
- 1/8 teaspoon of sea salt optional
- 50 grams (about 1/2 cup) of cocoa butter
- 1/2 cup of unsweetened cocoa; you can use Ghirardelli
- 1/4 cup of low-carb sugar substitute or 1 tablespoon plus 2 teaspoons of Trivia
- 1/4 teaspoon of almonds finely chopped, optional

PREPARATIONS

- In a double boiler or chocolate melter, melt cocoa butter.
- Stir in sweetener, salt, and cocoa powder.
- Keep on heat until the dry ingredients have been incorporated very well into the melted cocoa butter.
- Remove from the heat.
- Stir in chopped almonds and vanilla extract.
- Pour out on a chocolate mold or prepared pan.
- Sprinkle with chopped almonds and additional salt if you want.
- Serve and enjoy.

PREP TIME : 5 mins
COOK TIME : 15 mins
TOTAL TIME : 20 mins
YIELD : 10 pieces

GINGER CUPCAKES

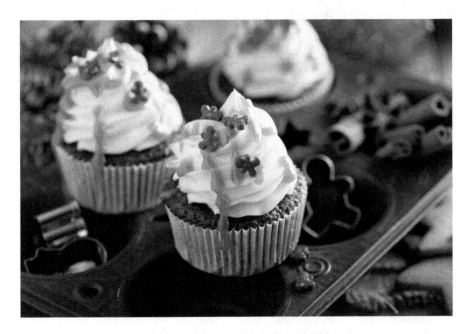

This Ginger Cupcake is one of my favorite holiday and diabetic recipes. It's warm and full of sweet spices.

You can enjoy this gluten-free treat all year long with whole wheat flour, egg whites, and unsweetened applesauce.

INGREDIENTS

- 1 cup of whole wheat flour
- 2 1/2 teaspoons of baking soda
- 1 teaspoon of ground ginger
- 1 teaspoon of ground allspice
- 1 teaspoon of ground cinnamon
- 1/2 cup of canola oil
- 2 egg whites
- 1 egg
- 2/3 cup of sugar
- 1 cup of molasses
- 1 cup of unsweetened applesauce
- 1 1/2 cup of all-purpose flour
- 1/2 teaspoon of salt
- 1 1/3 cup of reduced-fat frozen whipped topping, thawed

PREPARATIONS

- Preheat oven to 350 degrees F.
- Use paper liners to line muffin tins.
- Beat the egg whites, oil, egg and sugar until well blended in a large bowl.
- Add applesauce and molasses. Mix well.
- Combine flours, ginger, baking soda, cinnamon, allspice, and salt in a bowl.
- Beat in applesauce mixture gradually until blended.
- Spoon mixture into the muffin tins, filling each for about 2/3 full.
- Bake until a toothpick inserted in the center comes out clean, for about 18 to 22 minutes.
- Cool completely just before serving.
- Top each of the cupcake with 1 tablespoon of whipped topping.
- Serve and enjoy.

PREP TIME : 10 mins
COOK TIME : 22 mins
TOTAL TIME : 32 mins
YIELD : 24 cupcakes

BAKED CUSTARD

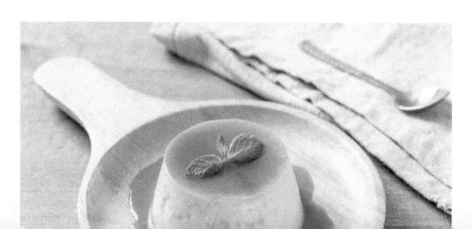

Do you know what I love about this recipe?

Baked Custard is so fantastic and easy to follow. You can add some nutmeg to the top before serving and top it with fresh, homemade whipped cream. Oh my goodness! So yummy!

You would want to make more and more of it even know though you didn't change anything in the recipe.

INGREDIENTS

- 1/4 teaspoon of ground nutmeg
- 1/4 teaspoon of ground cinnamon
- 3 teaspoons of vanilla extract
- 2-2/3 cups of whole milk
- 4 large eggs
- 2/3 cup of sugar
- 1/2 teaspoon of salt

PREPARATIONS

- Combine sugar, eggs, vanilla and spices in a bowl.
- Blend in milk and pour into a 1- and 1/2-quart baking dish.
- Place the baking dish inside a cake pan in the oven.
- Bake at 325 degrees until a knife inserted near the middle comes out clean, or for about an hour.
- Serve and enjoy.

PREP TIME : 10 mins
BAKE TIME : 6 mins
TOTAL TIME : 16 mins
YIELD : 6 servings

CHOCO MOUSSE

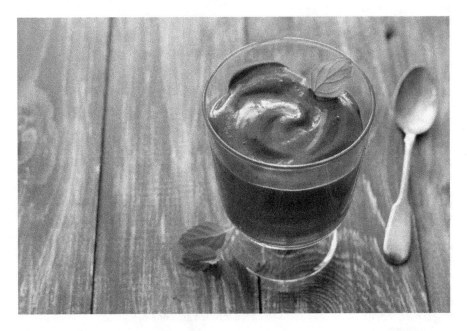

You won't imagine how good this will be until you give it a try!

This version of Chocolate Mousse is low carb and it will be so good. You can actually make a batch of it in a big bowl with the biggest serving spoon. It will be a knockout!

Is it Valentine's day already? Why not feel the love with this Chocolate Mousse using fancy glasses to serve? Smile!

INGREDIENTS

- 2 medium egg yolks
- 1/4 cup of granulated sugar substitute
- 1 teaspoon of pure vanilla extract
- 7 ounces (2 bars) of Perugina or Ghirardelli bittersweet or dark chocolate
- 2 tablespoons of strong coffee (you can use decaffeinated espresso)
- 2 tablespoons of orange liquor or Bourbon (optional)
- 3/4 cup plus 3 tablespoons of whipping cream
- 3 medium egg whites

PREPARATIONS

- Break up to 5 ounces of the chocolate.
- Place the chocolate, liquor and coffee in a small pot.
- In a larger pot of hot water that has been turned off the heat, cover and place the small pot and allow it to melt.
- Beat sugar substitute and egg yolks until frothy.
- Add the 3 tablespoons of whipping cream and vanilla into the egg mixture then beat to combine.
- Whisk the melted chocolate until shiny and smooth.
- Add the melted chocolate to the egg mixture slowly, stirring constantly.
- Beat egg whites until stiff peaks form.
- Fold in 1/4 of the egg whites into the chocolate to lighten the mixture.
- Fold in the rest of the egg whites.
- Grate about 2 ounces of chocolate on the medium side of a box grater. Fold into the mixture.
- Beat 3/4 cup of whipping cream until it holds its shape and triples in bulk.
- Fold the whipped cream into the rest of the mixture.
- Pour 6 glasses or into 1 large bowl.
- Chill for about 4 to 5 hours. Serve and enjoy.

PREP TIME : 25 mins
COOK TIME : 5 mins
TOTAL TIME : 30 mins
YIELD : 6 servings

CHRISTMAS COOKIES

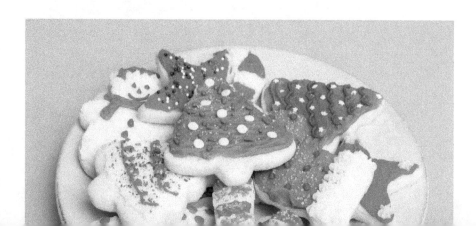

These cookies could be easily shared and given to neighbors and friends. These cookies always lead to a baking bonanza to prepare for Christmas.

You should try icing these cookies when cold. And before baking, make sure you sprinkle with colored sugar. They would be perfect, fantastic and beautiful.

INGREDIENTS

- 2 teaspoons of baking powder
- 1/2 cup of skim milk
- 2 tablespoons of water
- 1 teaspoon of vanilla extract
- 1/2 cup of shortening
- 3 tablespoons of sugar substitute
- 1 egg
- Several drops of food coloring (optional)
- 2 1/2 cups of cake flour
- 1/2 teaspoon of salt

PREPARATIONS

- Cream the shortening.
- Add egg, sweetener and food coloring; beat well.
- Combine dry ingredients in a separate bowl; add the vanilla, milk and water.
- Put in the flour mixture and stir well.
- Chill the dough for about 2 to 4 hours.
- Preheat oven to 325 degrees F.
- Roll out 1/8 inch thick and cut the cookies into your desired shapes.
- Bake for about 8 to 10 minutes.
- Cool and store in an air-tight container.
- Enjoy.

PREP TIME : 10 mins
CHILL TIME : 4 hours
TOTAL TIME : 4 hours 10 mins
YIELD : 24 servings

ECLAIR BITES

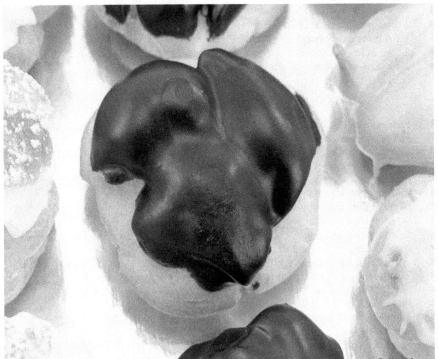

While desserts from the bakery aren't always the best option if you're following a diabetic diet, that does not mean you will never get to enjoy your favorites again.

With this recipe for Eclair Bites, you can savor the sweetness of a classic bakery treat without going overboard.

I hope you enjoy it.

INGREDIENTS

- 1 1/2 stick margarine, melted
- 1 (4-serving size) package sugar-free instant French vanilla pudding mix
- 1 1/4 cup of low-fat milk
- 2 cups of reduced-fat graham cracker crumbs
- 1/2 cup of confectioners' sugar
- 2 cups of fat-free frozen whipped topping, thawed
- 3/4 cup of sugar-free chocolate frosting

PREPARATIONS

- Preheat oven to 350 degrees F.
- Use paper liners to line 18 mini muffin cups.
- Combine together sugar, graham crackers, and butter in a medium bowl; mix well.
- Press mixture evenly into paper liners.
- Press over the bottom and up sides of liners using your fingers.
- Bake until crust starts to brown or for about 5 minutes.
- Remove from the oven and leave to completely cool.
- Whisk pudding mixture and milk in a medium bowl.
- Fold in whipped topping.
- Place in a plastic bag and snip off one corner.
- Fill your graham cracker crusts evenly with pudding mixture.
- Heat frosting for about 10 to 15 seconds in a small microwave safe bowl.
- Stir until pourable and smooth.
- Place in a plastic bag and snip off one corner.
- Top pudding mixture with 1 dollop of chocolate frosting.
- Refrigerate until ready to serve, for about 4 hours.
- Serve and enjoy.

COOK TIME : 5 mins
CHILL TIME : 4 hours
TOTAL TIME : 4 hours 10 mins
YIELD : 18 servings

SNICKER DOODLES

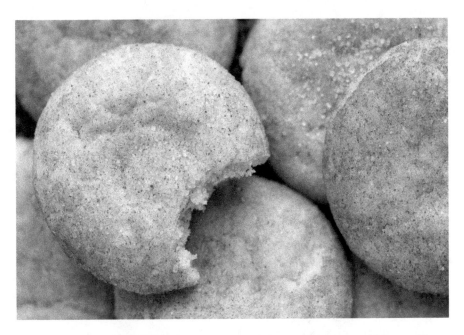

Due to my taste, I added extra vanilla, and it felt good. You can add it too, if you truly want the full experience.

You'll be needing a little cinnamon on the rolling sugar to get that beautiful cinnamon coating. Snickerdoodles taste delicious and they are easy to make.

This might be your first-time making snickerdoodles, but I promise you that it's definitely going to work out great!

Enjoy.

INGREDIENTS

- 1-1/2 cups of all-purpose flour
- 1/4 teaspoon of baking soda
- 1/4 teaspoon of cream of tartar
- 1 teaspoon of ground cinnamon
- 1/2 cup of softened butter
- 1 cup plus 2 tablespoons of sugar, divided
- 1 large egg, room temperature
- 1/2 teaspoon of vanilla extract

PREPARATIONS

- Preheat oven to 375 degrees F.
- Cream butter and 1 cup of sugar until fluffy and light.
- Beat in vanilla and egg.
- Whisk together baking soda, flour and cream of tartar in a separate bowl.
- Gradually beat into creamed mixture.
- Mix the rest of the sugar and cinnamon in small bowl.
- Shape dough into 1-inch balls.
- Roll in cinnamon sugar.
- Place 2-inches apart on ungreased baking sheets.
- Bake for about 10 to 12 minutes, until light browned.
- Remove from pans to wire racks to cool.
- Serve and enjoy.

PREP TIME : 20 mins
BAKE TIME : 10 mins
TOTAL TIME : 30 mins
YIELD : 2 and 1/2 dozen

LEMON BARS

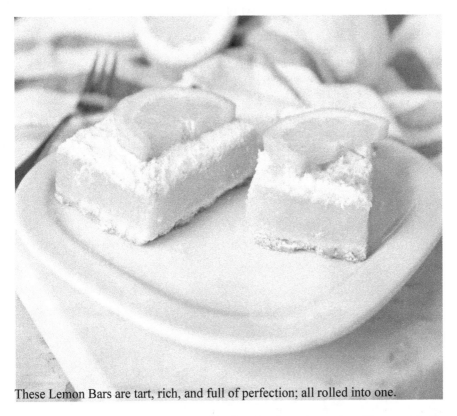

These Lemon Bars are tart, rich, and full of perfection; all rolled into one.

Put a smile on your friend's faces with this simple recipe today. The crust is the perfect thickness, and there is enough lemon custard in each bite to satisfy them.

This recipe makes a lot of crust and spreads into a 9 by 13 dish easily but makes a thinner bar. Make sure to increase the cooking time of the crust and fill an extra 5 to 10 minutes each if you'll be using a smaller baking dish, which is 8 by 11.

INGREDIENTS

- 4 eggs
- 1 and 1/2 cups of white sugar
- 1/4 cup of all-purpose flour
- 1 cup of butter, softened
- 1/2 cup of white sugar
- 2 cups of all-purpose flour
- 2 lemons, juiced

- Preheat oven to 350 degrees F.
- Blend together softened butter, 1/2 cup of sugar and 2 cups of flours in a medium bowl.
- Press into the bottom of an ungreased 9 by 13-inch pan.
- Bake in the preheated oven, for about 15 to 20 minutes, or until golden and firm.
- Whisk together the rest of the sugar and 1/4 cup of flour in a separate bowl.
- Whisk in the lemon juice and eggs.
- Pour over the baked crust.
- Bake for another 20 minutes in the preheated oven.
- The bars will firm up as they cool. Make another pan using limes instead of lemons for a festive tray, adding drops of green food coloring.
- After both pans have cooled, cut 2 into uniform 2-inch squares and arrange in a checkerboard fashion.
- Serve and enjoy.

PREP TIME : 15 mins
BAKE TIME : 40 mins
TOTAL TIME : 55 mins
YIELD : 36 servings

UPSIDE DOWN PINEAPPLE CAKE

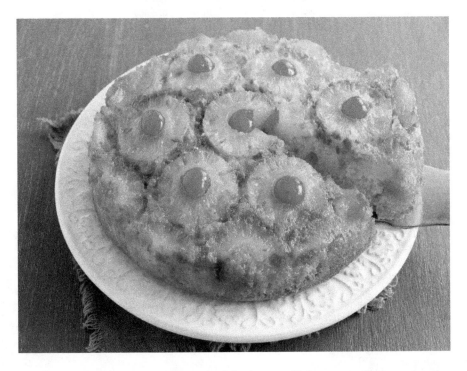

This Classic Upside-Down Pineapple Cake boasts all the gooey, fruity, caramel-y goodness made for generations and generations to come - in addition to a secret shortcut so you can make it in a snap.

With your yellow cake mix, you can have this impressive dessert prepped for the oven within 15 minutes.

All you need to do is bake, flip, and bring to the table to add a colorful and sweet flourish to any party. Enjoy.

- 1 can (20 ounces) of pineapple slices in juice, drained, juice reserved
- 1 jar (6 ounces) of maraschino cherries without stems, drained
- 1 box of yellow cake mix
- 1/4 cup of butter
- 1 cup of packed brown sugar
- Vegetable oil and eggs called for on cake mix box

PREPARATIONS

- Heat oven to 350 degrees F.
- Melt butter in the oven in 13 by 9-inch pan.
- Sprinkle brown sugar over butter.
- Arrange pineapples slices on brown sugar.
- In the center of each pineapple slice, place a cherry and arrange remaining cherries around slices; gently press into brown sugar.
- Add enough water into the reserved pineapple juice to measure 1 cup.
- Make your batter, substituting pineapple juice mixture for the water.
- Pour batter over cherries and pineapple.
- Bake for about 45 minutes or until toothpick inserted in center comes out clean.
- Loosen cake by running knife around side of the pan.
- Place your heatproof serving plate upside down onto a pan. turn the plate and pan over.
- Now, leave for just 5 minutes so the brown sugar topping can drizzle over cake.
- Remove pan and cool for about 30 minutes.
- Serve cool or warm.
- Enjoy.

PREP TIME : 15 mins
BAKE TIME : 1 hour 35 mins
TOTAL TIME : 1 hour 50 mins
YIELD : 12 servings

CARROT CAKE TOWERS

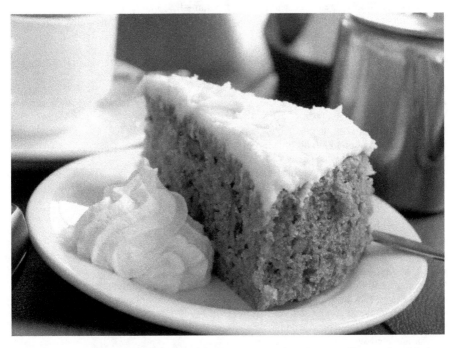

You don't have to be diabetic to enjoy this carrot cake. Carrot cake can be good or really, really bad, and this recipe has a flax-seed meal. But nothing could be further from the truth. This cake is super delicious and by adding the cream cheese, the frosting is divine.

These would be perfect for a party and it's a recipe you can make over and over again. They can be made into squares and triangles - it's your choice.

INGREDIENTS

- 1/4 teaspoon of salt
- 3 cups of finely shredded carrot about 6 medium-size (3 large for me)
- 1 cup of refrigerated or frozen egg product thawed, or 4 eggs, lightly beaten
- 1/2 cup of granulated sugar or sugar substitute blend-equivalent to 1/2 cup of granulated sugar
- 1/2 cup of packed brown sugar or brown sugar substitute blend-equivalent to 1/2 cup of brown sugar
- 1/2 cup of canola oil
- 1 1/2 cups of all-purpose flour
- 2/3 cup of flax seed meal
- 2 teaspoons of baking powder
- 1 teaspoon of pumpkin pie spice
- 1/2 teaspoon of baking soda
- 1 recipe of Fluffy Cream Cheese Frosting
- Coarsely shredded carrot optional

PREPARATIONS

- Preheat oven to 350 degrees F.
- Grease the bottom of a baking pan.
- Use waxed paper to line bottom of pan.
- Grease and flour the waxed paper and the sides of the pan lightly; set it aside.
- In a large bowl, stir together flax seed meal, flour, baking powder, baking soda, pumpkin pie spice, and salt; set it aside.
- In a separate large bowl, combine eggs, finely shredded carrot, brown sugar, granulated sugar and oil.
- Add egg mixture all at once into the flour mixture. Stir until well combined.
- Spoon batter into prepared pan, spreading evenly.
- Bake until a toothpick inserted near the center comes out clean, or for about 25 minutes.
- Cool cake in pan on a wire rack for about 10 minutes.
- Invert cake onto a wire rack and cool completely.
- Transfer cake onto a large cutting board.
- Make cutouts in the cake using a 2-inch round cutter, leaving as little space between the cutouts (you'd get 29 to 33 cutouts)
- For each of the servings, place one of the cake cutouts on a serving plate.
- Spread about 1 tablespoon of fluffy cream cheese frosting on top of the cake round.
- If desired, garnish with coarsely carrot, shredded.
- Serve and enjoy.

PREP TIME : 15 mins
BAKE TIME : 25 mins
TOTAL TIME : 50 mins
YIELD : 16 servings

GUMMY WORMS

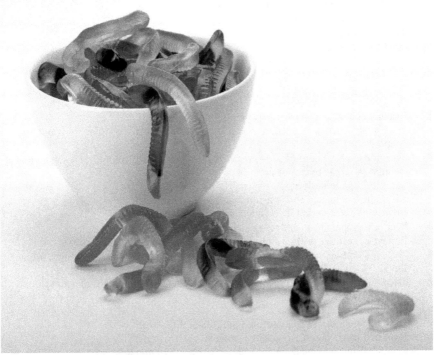

This recipe makes dual-flavored raspberry and orange worms.

You can substitute other juices to change the flavors. You can as well make with a single flavor. Your kids would love it.

- 12 tablespoons of sugar (separated)
- 8 tablespoons of corn syrup (separated)
- 2/3 cup of orange juice
- 8 tablespoons of unflavored gelatin (separated)
- 1/2 cup of cold water (divided)
- 2/3 cup of raspberry juice
- Optional: food coloring

PREPARATIONS

- Bring together all the ingredients.
- Prepare an 8 by 8-inch pan by using water to wet it.
- Place 4 tablespoons of gelatin inside a 1/4 cup of cold water to soften for about 5 minutes.
- Place the 6 tablespoons of sugar, raspberry juice, and 4 tablespoons of corn syrup in a medium saucepan over medium heat.
- Stir until sugar dissolves.
- Stir in the gelatin and continue until the gelatin dissolves.
- Now, add food coloring if you'll be using it.
- Pour into prepared pan and refrigerate until set, for about an hour.
- **Repeat procedure with orange juice by:**
- Placing 4 tablespoons of gelatin in 1/4 cup of cold water for about 5 minutes, to soften.
- Place the 6 tablespoons of sugar, raspberry juice, and 4 tablespoons of corn syrup in a medium saucepan over medium heat.
- Stir until sugar dissolves.
- Stir in the gelatin and continue until the gelatin dissolves.
- Now, add food coloring if you'll be using it.
- Remove from heat and allow it to cool in a pan for 10 minutes.
- Pour over raspberry layer and refrigerate until set, for an hour.
- Turn out of the pan when set and cut with a sharp knife into long, thin strips to resemble worms.
- Enjoy.

PREP TIME : 10 mins
COOL TIME : 20 mins
TOTAL TIME : 30 mins
YIELD : 8 servings

PUMPKIN PIE

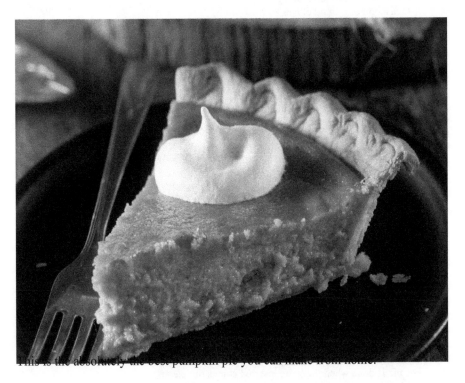

This is the absolutely the best pumpkin pie you can make from home.

Make it with fresh or canned pumpkin puree, and up to several days ahead.

I love this pie because they freeze well and it can be called the "Thanksgiving pie." But real Thanksgiving pie never looks so good and easy like that. I am in love with this recipe already. I hope you love it too.

- 1/4 teaspoon of ground nutmeg
- 1/4 teaspoon of ground cloves
- 1/8 teaspoon of ground cardamom
- 1/2 teaspoon of lemon zest
- 2 cups of pumpkin pulp purée from a sugar pumpkin OR 1 15-ounce can of pumpkin purée (can also use puréed cooked butternut squash)
- 1 1/2 cup of heavy cream or one 12 ounces can of evaporated milk
- 2 large eggs plus the yolk of a third egg
- 1/2 cup of packed dark brown sugar
- 1/3 cup of white sugar
- 1/2 teaspoon of salt
- 2 teaspoons of cinnamon
- 1 teaspoon of ground ginger
- 1 good pie crust, chilled or frozen

PREPARATIONS

- Preheat your oven to 425 degrees F.
- In a large bowl, beat the eggs.
- Mix in the white sugar, brown sugar, cinnamon, salt, nutmeg, ground ginger, lemon zest, ground cloves and cardamom.
- Mix in the pumpkin puree.
- Stir in the cream and beat till everything is well combined.
- Pour the filling into a frozen pie shell.
- Bake at high temperature for 15 minutes at 425 degrees F.
- Lower the temperature to 350 degrees F after 15 minutes.
- Bake for about 45 to 55 minutes more.
- The pie is done when the knife inserted comes out clean.
- Cool the pumpkin pie on a wire rack for about 2 hours.
- Top with whipped cream
- Serve and enjoy.

PREP TIME : 20 mins
COOL TIME : 1 hour
TOTAL TIME : 1 hour 20 mins
YIELD : 8 servings

ALMOND MACAROONS

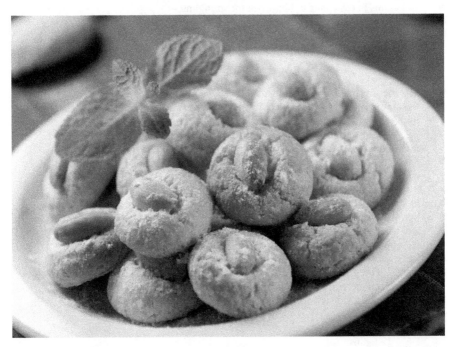

This recipe is the best for creating marvelous almond macaroons at home. The outsides are crisp and they are traditionally baked on edible rice paper; this is because they are extremely difficult to remove from the baking tray.

By the way, you can have some fun with fillings and flavors with these homemade almond macaroons. Enjoy.

INGREDIENTS

- 225 grams of ground almonds
- 200 grams of caster sugar, plus extra for sprinkling.
- 3 medium free-range egg whites.
- 15 whole blanched almonds split into half lengthways.

PREPARATIONS

- Mix the sugar and ground almonds into a large mixing bowl.
- Beat the egg whites with an electric mixer in a separate bowl on a slow speed until just frothy.
- Add the egg whites into the sugar and almonds, 1 tablespoon at a time, mixing after each spoonful.
- Keep going until the mixture is soft and not runny. You might need to use all the egg whites.
- Roll the mix into walnut size balls and space them apart on the baking trays.
- Flatten them slightly by pressing a blanched almond half into the top of each one.
- Sprinkle some caster sugar over the top of each, then leave them for about 10 to 15 minutes to sit.
- Heat the oven to 190 degrees C.
- Bake until pale golden brown, for about 15 to 20 minutes.
- Leave on the baking sheet for at least 10 minutes before transferring to a cooling rack to cool completely. They'll get harden as they cool.
- Serve with a cuppa.
- Enjoy.

PREP TIME : 20 mins
COOL TIME : 20 mins
TOTAL TIME : 40 mins
YIELD : 30 macaroons

CHOCO THICK COOKIES

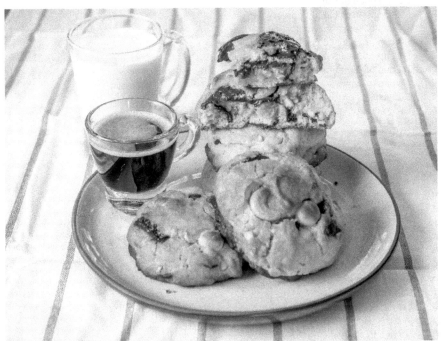

These cookies are golden and beautiful on the outside, gooey and soft on the inside. It is loaded up with tons of melted chocolate.

The best thing about these cookies is their size. These cookies are hearty, thick, chewy, buttery, and extremely loaded with chocolate.

I hope you'll enjoy it.

- 2 cups of all-purpose flour
- 1/2 teaspoon of salt
- 1/2 teaspoon of baking powder
- 3/4 cup of semi-sweet chocolate chips
- 1/4 cup of chopped pecans
- 1/2 cup of unsalted butter, room temperature
- 3/4 cup of light brown sugar
- 1/4 cup of white sugar
- 1 large egg
- 1 teaspoon of vanilla extract

PREPARATIONS

- Use a silicone baking mat to line a large baking sheet; set it aside.
- Add the sugars and butter in a large mixing bowl.
- Cream the butter and sugars using a stand mixer or a hand together until fluffy.
- Add in the vanilla, large egg, then mix until combined.
- Add the baking powder, flour, and salt.
- Mix until well combined. The dough might seem to be crumbling.
- Pour in the pecans and chocolate chips and mix them using your hands.
- Divide the dough into 6 pieces.
- Gently form into a cookie shape and place on the baking sheet.
- Bake the cookies until golden brown, or for about 18 minutes.
- Let the cookies cool on the baking sheet for at 5 minutes, then remove to a wire rack to continue cooling.
- Serve and enjoy.

PREP TIME : 10 mins
COOK TIME : 16 mins
CHILL TIME : 30 mins
TOTAL TIME : 56 mins
YIELD : 6 servings

POACHED PEARS

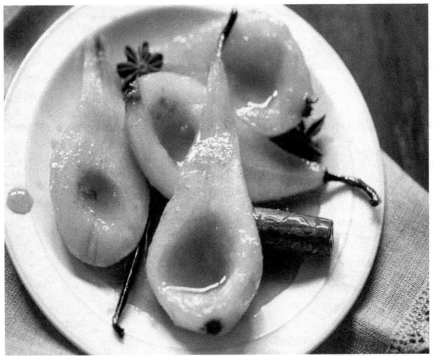

Your Poached Pears can be served with some mascarpone cheese, a scoop of vanilla ice cream, or whipped cream for an impressive diabetic dessert.

It's an easy and simple recipe that is absolutely elegant. They have a great balance of spice, sweet and fruity flavors.

It's mildly sweet and crisp making them the perfect canvas for all the flavors in the poaching liquid.

INGREDIENTS

- 1 teaspoon of ground nutmeg
- 4 whole pears
- 1/2 cup of fresh raspberries
- 1 cup of orange juice
- 1/4 cup of apple juice
- 1 teaspoon of ground cinnamon
- 2 tablespoons of orange zest

PREPARATIONS

- Mix together apple juice, orange juice, nutmeg, and ground cinnamon in a small bowl.
- Stir ingredients until well mixed; set it aside.
- Peel the pears and leave the stems.
- Remove the core from the bottom of the pear and in a shallow saucepan, place the pears.
- Pour over juice mixture into the pan and set over medium heat.
- Simmer your pears for about 30 minutes, turning frequently.
- Don't bring liquid to a boil.
- Transfer the pears to individual plates.
- Garnish with orange zest and raspberries.
- Serve immediately and enjoy.

PREP TIME : 10 mins
COOK TIME : 30 mins
TOTAL TIME : 40 mins
YIELD : 4 servings

PUMPKIN MOUSSE

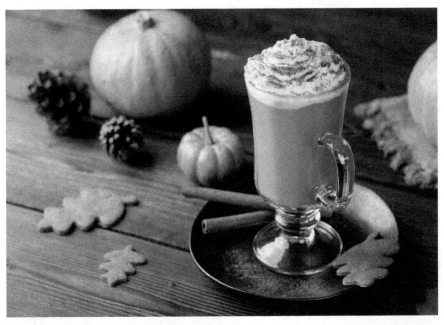

Pumpkin mousse is fluffy, creamy, melt in your mouth perfection, and it is one of my family's favorite pumpkin desserts.

When I make it every year, another die-heard pumpkin-hater falls prey to its awesomeness. You need to give it a try!

INGREDIENTS

- 2 tablespoons of maple syrup
- 1/2 teaspoon of pure vanilla extract
- 1 cup of whole milk
- 1 1/2 cup of heavy cream
- 1 (3.4 ounces) package of instant vanilla pudding
- 1 teaspoon of pumpkin spice
- 1/2 teaspoon of cinnamon, plus more for garnish
- 1/2 teaspoon of kosher salt
- 1 (15-ounces) can of pumpkin purée

PREPARATIONS

- Whisk together spices, pudding mix and salt in a large bowl.
- Add maple syrup, vanilla, pumpkin, and whole milk, then beat until smooth with a hand mixer.
- Whip heavy cream for about 3 to 4 minutes, until stiff peaks form in another large bowl.
- Fold 2/3 of the whipped cream into the pumpkin mixture until smooth.
- Spoon into serving dishes.
- Top with the remaining whipped cream.
- Garnish with a sprinkle of cinnamon.
- Serve and enjoy.

PREP TIME : 10 mins
COOK TIME : 0 mins
TOTAL TIME : 10 mins
YIELD : 4 servings

YOGURT BLUEBERRY POPSICLES

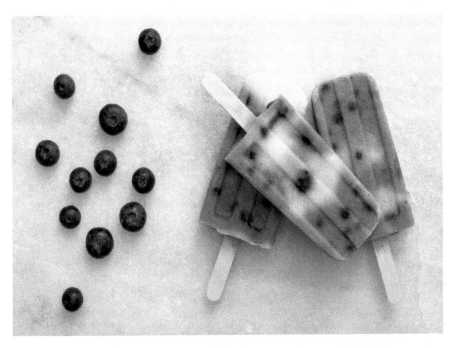

Yogurt Blueberry Popsicles are made with protein-packed three (3) ingredients that are so healthy for the body.

These popsicles hit the spot when the weather heats up. It's a diabetic and gluten-free treat you need to try today.

INGREDIENTS

- 2 cups of blueberries
- 2 tablespoons of honey or agave
- 2 cups of vanilla Greek yogurt or any flavor of your choice

PREPARATIONS

- In a food processor or blender, blend the blueberries on high speed until nearly liquified into a smoothie.
- In a large bowl, pour the thick blueberry liquid.
- Stir in the honey/agave.
- Add the yogurt and gently mix everything together.
- For a swirly look for your popsicles - do not fully blend the blueberries and yogurt.
- The mixture will be thick. Now, taste it and if you want it sweeter, you can add a little more honey/agave.
- Pour the mixture evenly into each of the popsicle molds.
- You can insert them before freezing if your popsicle mold has slots for sticks. If not, freeze for about 2 hours.
- Put a wooden popsicle stick in the middle.
- Continue to freeze for an additional 5 hours or over the night.
- Run the popsicle molds under warm water to remove easily.
- Eat on a hot day.
- Serve and enjoy.

PREP TIME : 10 mins
COOK TIME : 0 mins
TOTAL TIME : 6 to 8 hours
YIELD : 6 popsicles

LEMON PIE CURD

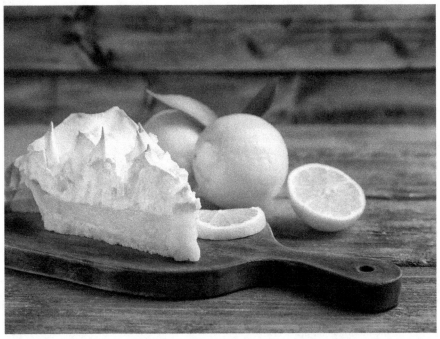

Lemon Pie Curd is a delicious dessert packed with coconut flour pie crust and sugar-free lemon curd. It's 100% paleo, keto, and gluten-free.

This recipe is perfect when served with sugar-free meringue and strawberries. I have tested this recipe before and I love it so much. You should add it to your favorites - so healthy.

- 1 coconut flour pie crust
- Sugar Free Lemon Pie Curd
- 2 Egg Yolk - keep egg white for meringue
- 1/2 cup of Butter or coconut oil, melted
- 1/2 cup of Lemon Juice or juice of about 5 small lemons
- 2 Eggs
- 1/4 cup of Erythritol - erythritol or monk fruit sugar
- Sugar Free Meringue Frosting
- 2 egg whites
- 1/4 cup of Erythritol

PREPARATIONS

- Prepare your Coconut Flour Pie Crust
  Preparing the Lemon Pie Curd:
- In a saucepan, whisk the lemon juice, eggs, sweetener, and egg yolks together.
- Bring to a medium heat and add the butter or coconut oil, stirring continuously to prevent the eggs from scrambling and cooking.
- Increase the heat to medium high when the coconut oil is melted, keep stirring until it thickens up.
- Remove from heat and transfer into a bowl to cool down at room temperature for about 15 minutes.
- Fill in the coconut flour pie crust with the lemon pie curd.
- Refrigerate the lemon pie to firm up for at least 2 hours.
  Preparing the Meringue Frosting:
- Add the meringue before serving.
- Whisk the egg whites in a bowl until it starts producing a good volume.
- This is usually 30 seconds on high speed.
- Keep whisking on high speed and add the sugar free crystal sweetener of your choice slowly.
- After 1 minute, the meringue should be really fluffy and triple its volume.
- Tip the bowl upside down to check if the meringue is ready.
- Transfer on the top of the lemon pie curd if it sticks to the bowl.
- Torch the top of the meringue or place for 2 minutes in the oven or grill more until the top is brown slightly.
- Serve and enjoy.

PREP TIME : 20 mins
COOK TIME : 20 mins
TOTAL TIME : 40 mins
YIELD : 8 servings

BOUNTY BARS

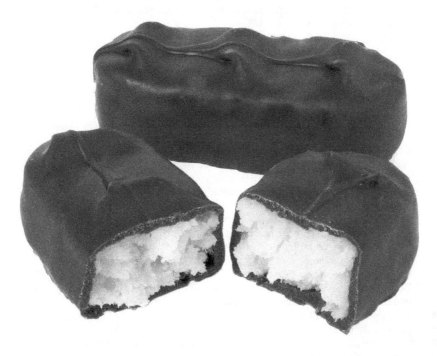

Bounty bars are healthy, raw homemade candy bars that are 100% keto, paleo, sugar-free, and diabetic friendly.

This recipe can be made within 30 minutes, with only four ingredients. The bars are mainly made of healthy fats from coconut oil. These bars do not contain many calories and they are very filling.

You can adjust the sweetness with extra stevia drops if you have a really sweet tooth.

INGREDIENTS

- 2 cups of unsweetened desiccated coconut
- 1/3 cup of Coconut oil, melted, at room temperature
- Half cup of Canned Coconut cream, shake the can before use, full-fat minimum 30% fat, at room temperature (not cold)
- 1/3 cup of Erythritol
- **Chocolate Coating:**
- 6 ounces of Sugar-free Chocolate Chips
- 2 teaspoon of Coconut oil
- 1-2 Monk Fruit Drops or Stevia Drops

PREPARATIONS

- Cover a square 9 by 9 inch pan with parchment paper and set it aside.
- Add melted coconut oil, erythritol, desiccated coconut and canned coconut cream in a food processor.
- Process on high speed, for at least 1 minute.
- You may have to process for 20 seconds. Stop and scrape down the bowl and repeat until it comes together into a fine wet coconut batter.
- Press the raw dough onto the prepared pan.
- Make sure there's no air left between the batter.
- Use your hands to press the batter and use spatula to flatten the surface.
- Freeze for 10 minutes to firm up.
- Don't freeze them too long or they might get so much hard as it's difficult to cut them into bars - they might break into pieces.
- But they will still look delicious and less pretty.
- Remove from the freezer.
- Lift up the parchment paper to release the coconut block from the pan.
- Place on a chopping board.
- Cut into 20 rectangles using a sharp knife.
- Shape each rectangle into your hands to form round borders like the real Bounty Bar if you want.
- Place each formed bounty bars on plate covered with parchment paper.
- Set it aside in the freezer while you prepare the chocolate coating.
- Meanwhile, in the microwave, melt the sugar free chocolate chips with coconut oil.
- Microwave until fully melted by 30 seconds.
- Add stevia drops to adjust sweetness to your taste if you want.
- Dip each coconut bar into the melted chocolate mixture using 2 forks.
- Freeze again to set the chocolate shell when all the bars have been covered with chocolate.
- Store the bounty bars in the fridge in an airtight container for up to a month or freeze.
- Defrost for about half hour before eating.
- Serve and enjoy.

PREP TIME : 10 mins
COOK TIME : 0 mins
TOTAL TIME : 30 mins
YIELD : 20 bars

COTTAGE CHEESE

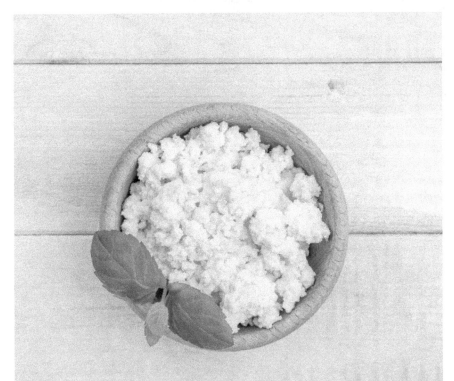

What I love about Cottage Cheese is the flavor. It always makes my day. This recipe is a must-have at any family potluck, church, dinner, or holiday gatherings. You can pretty much use any Jell-o you prefer. It's just as good with just about any.

You can also add chopped pecans for texture if you want.

Enjoy!

INGREDIENTS

- 3 cups of low-fat cottage cheese
- 2 (0.3 ounces) packages of sugar-free lemon-flavored Jell-O mix
- 1 (8 ounces) container of lite frozen whipped topping, thawed

PREPARATIONS

- In a food processor, place the cottage cheese and blend until creamy.
- Whisk in the flavored gelatin powder.
- Fold in the thawed whipped topping.
- Refrigerate until serving.
- Serve and enjoy.

PREP TIME : 5 mins
ADDITIONAL TIME : 30 mins
TOTAL TIME : 35 mins
YIELD : 6 servings

BERRY COBBLER

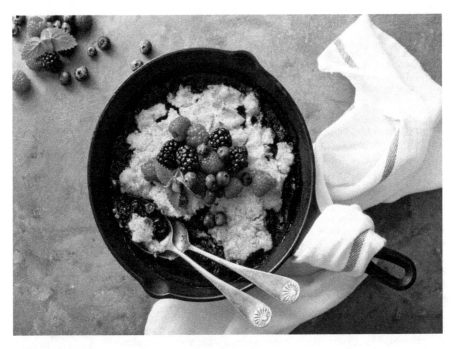

This classic dessert has zero sugar added so all the sweetness comes from the berries themselves. *Smile* - you would love them!

You can choose your favorite berries to put into this berry cobbler recipe. It's up to you.

Filling:
- 3 tablespoons of cornstarch
- 4 cups of blackberries or marionberries, boysenberries, blueberries
- 1 packet of sweetener up to 2 packets, as sweet as 2 teaspoons of sugar each, optional
- 3 tablespoons of water
- 1/2 cup of fruit-sweet boysenberry syrup or blueberry syrup
- 3/4 teaspoon of cinnamon

Dough:
- 1 cup of unbleached flour
- 2 tablespoons of apple juice concentrate
- 1/4 cup of low-fat fruit-sweet berry yogurt or cherry flavor
- 1 and 1/2 teaspoon of baking powder
- 1/2 teaspoon of salt
- 2 tablespoons of butter, melted

PREPARATIONS

- Preheat the oven to 400 degrees F.
- Use nonstick spray to cover a deep-dish pie pan.

Making the filling:
- Stir cornstarch into the water until dissolved.
- Mix in cinnamon and syrup.
- Let it sit and set it aside.

Making the dough:
- Sift together baking powder, flour and salt.
- Combine juice concentrate, butter and yogurt in a separate bowl.
- Pour wet ingredients over the dry ingredients.
- Gently blend with a fork for about 20 to 30 seconds.
- Knead the dough for about 20 to 30 more seconds.
- Press dough into approximately 1/4 to 1/2 inch thickness on a floured surface and wide enough to cover your pan.

Making the pie:
- Fold rinsed, drained berries into filling mixture.
- Pour berry filling into a greased pan.
- Over the top, set the cobbler dough, making the dough surface as even as possible.
- Press the dough against the sides of the pan.
- Cut a design in the dough for air ventilation.
- Turn oven down to 375 degrees F.
- Bake until the dough is light brown, or for about 20 to 25 minutes.
- Let it cool and serve.
- Enjoy.

PREP TIME : 15 mins
COOK TIME : 25 mins
TOTAL TIME : 40 mins
YIELD : 8 servings

CHOCO BANANA BITES

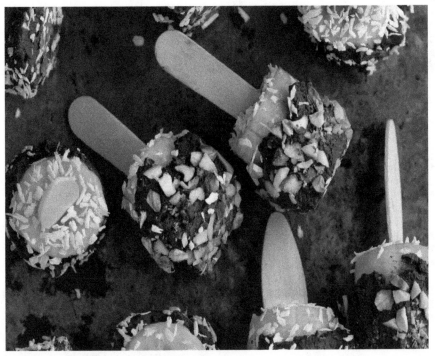

Choco Banana Bites are super easy to make and always a hit with everyone. They are so delicious - they taste like a treat!

And they are made with wholesome ingredients; they are refreshing, convenient, and very easy to make. You just need to grab a bite from the freezer whenever you need it and it's pretty hot on the outside.

You would love it!

INGREDIENTS

- 3 small (about 6-inches long) ripe bananas, each cut into 6 (1-inch.) slices
- 18 cocktail picks
- 2 tablespoons of unsweetened shredded dried coconut, toasted
- 2 tablespoons of chopped toasted almonds
- 1/2 teaspoon of sea salt flakes (such as Maldon)
- 5 ounces (85% cacao) of dark chocolate, finely chopped
- 2 teaspoons of coconut oil

PREPARATIONS

- Skewer each banana slice with 1 cocktail pick and place it on a parchment lined baking sheet.
- Freeze for an hour.
- Pour water into a depth of 1-inch bottom of a double boiler and set over medium heat; bring to a boil.
- Reduce heat to medium-low, then simmer.
- Place oil and chocolate in top of the double boiler and cook, turning often, until mixture is smooth and chocolate melts, or for about 4 minutes.
- In the chocolate mixture, dip 1 skewered banana slice.
- Sprinkle immediately with a pinch of coconut and return to a baking sheet.
- Repeat procedure with the rest of the coconut for 5 extra banana slices and almonds for 6 banana slices.
- Then with the sea salt for the remaining 6 banana slices.
- Freeze bites before serving, or for about an hour.
- Serve and enjoy.

PREP TIME : 12 mins
COOK TIME : 0 mins
TOTAL TIME : 2 hour 12 mins
YIELD : 18 bites

FIG ORANGE PIE

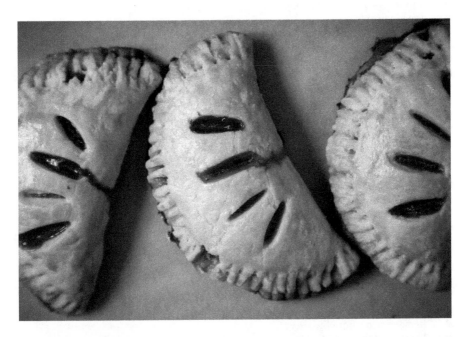

Fig orange pies are perfect for brunch gatherings, a sweet treat with your afternoon tea, and a diabetic-friendly dessert.

You just have to pick up one of these fruit-filled pastries and bite in. You would fall in love with this; it's pretty satisfying.

Enjoy!

- 1 cup all-purpose flour
- 3 fresh figs or 8 dried Mission figs
- 1 medium orange
- 1/4 cup of low-sugar orange marmalade
- Fat-free milk
- 1 teaspoon of powdered sugar
- 1/4 cup white whole-wheat flour or whole-wheat flour
- 2 tablespoons flax-seed meal
- 1/4 teaspoon salt
- 1/3 cup 60% to 70% tub-style vegetable oil spread, chilled
- 3-4 tablespoons cold water, divided

PREPARATIONS

- Preheat oven to 400 degrees F.
- Use parchment paper to line a large baking sheet; set it aside.
- Stir together flax-seeds meal, flours and salt in a medium bowl.
- Cut in chilled vegetable oil spread until pieces are pea size using a pastry blender.
- Sprinkle 1 tablespoon of cold water over part of the flour mixture. toss with a fork gently.
- Push moistened dough to the side of the bowl.
- Repeat moistening the flour mixture using 1 tablespoon of cold water at a time, until all the flour mixture is moistened.
- Divide the dough into 8 equal portions.
- Remove stems from figs.
- Place dried figs in a small bowl with enough boiling water to cover if you'll be using dried figs; let it stand for about 5 minutes to rehydrate, and then drain well.
- Chop the fresh or rehydrated dried figs.
- Shred enough orange peel to make 1/4 teaspoon and set it aside.
- Peel and chop the sections.
- Combine the chopped orange, figs, marmalade, and the shredded orange peel in a medium bowl. Stir well until combined.
- Roll each portion of the pastry dough on a lightly floured surface into 4-inch circle.
- Spoon the fig mixture atop the dough circles.
- Spread to an even layer, leave a 3/4-inch border on the edges.
- Moisten the edges of the dough circles using a little water.
- Fold the dough circles in half to make semi-circles.
- Press the edges to seal using the tines of a fork.
- Place the pies 2-inches apart on the prepared baking sheet.
- Make small slashes on the top of the pies to allow the steam to escape.
- Brush with milk lightly.
- Bake until the tops are golden brown, or for about 17 to 20 minutes.
- Transfer onto a wire rack. Cool for about 15 minutes.
- Sprinkle with powdered sugar lightly.
- Serve and enjoy.

PREP TIME : 40 mins
ADDITIONAL TIME : 0 mins
TOTAL TIME : 1 hour

YIELD : 8 servings

MICROWAVE POPCORN

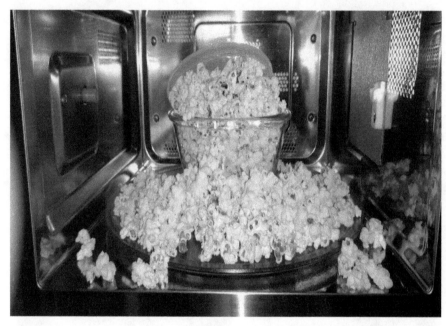

What I love about this Microwave Popcorn is that it's perfect for when it's chilly outside. It's packed with cocoa. If you are a fan of cocoa, you should have an interest in trying this recipe.

Enjoy the best two spectacular snacks with this delicately sweetened popcorn treat made inside the microwave.

Enjoy.

- 1/2 teaspoon of cocoa powder
- 1/2 teaspoon of sugar
- Pinch of salt
- 1 and 1/2 tablespoons of popcorn kernels
- 1/2 teaspoon of coconut oil

PREPARATIONS

- Add popcorn kernels to a brown paper bag.
- Fold the top of the bag over 3 times.
- Microwave for about 1 and half minutes, or until the popping stops.
- In a small microwave-safe bowl, place coconut oil and microwave for about 20 seconds, until melted. Stir with a fork.
- Add the cocoa powder, oil, salt, and sugar to the bag over the popped popcorn.
- Fold the top of the bag.
- Hold closed and shake to coat.
- Serve and enjoy.

PREP TIME : 5 mins
ADDITIONAL TIME : 0 mins
TOTAL TIME : 5 mins
YIELD : 1 serving

BLOSSOM COOKIES WITH PEANUT BUTTER

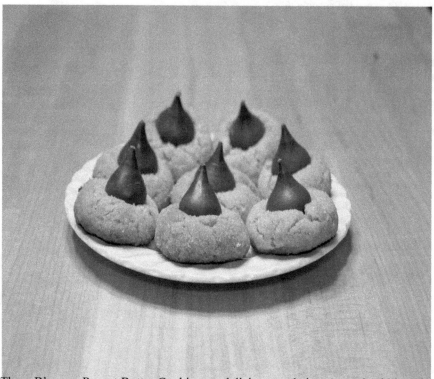

These Blossom Peanut Butter Cookies are delicious on their own—a healthier take on the best Christmas cookies around.

You can make them better by pressing a piece of dark chocolate candy into each of the hot cookies immediately after the cookies come out of the oven.

So yummy!

INGREDIENTS

- 1 cup of all-purpose flour
- 1/3 cup of whole-wheat flour
- 1/2 teaspoon of baking powder
- 1/2 teaspoon of baking soda
- 1/4 teaspoon of salt
- 1 cup of packed light brown sugar
- 1/4 cup of natural peanut butter
- 2 tablespoons of canola oil
- 1 large egg
- 1 teaspoon of vanilla extract
- 1 tablespoon of water
- 28 large dark chocolate candy pieces, unwrapped

PREPARATIONS

- Preheat oven to 350 degrees F.
- Use cooking spray to coat 2 baking sheets.
- Combine peanut butter, brown sugar, egg, oil and vanilla in a mixing bowl.
- Add water and beat until smooth with an electric mixer.
- Stir together whole-wheat flours and all-purpose, baking soda and salt in a small bowl.
- Stir the dry ingredients into the brown sugar mixture until well combined.
- Roll the dough between your palms into balls using wet hands and 1 tablespoon for each.
- Flatten each ball into half-inch thick dish.
- Place 2 inches apart on the prepared baking sheets.
- Bake the cookies, one sheet at a time for about 8 to 9 minutes, until golden.
- Press a chocolate piece immediately into each cookie's center.
- Transfer onto a wire rack to cool. Serve and enjoy.

PREP TIME : 30 mins
ADDITIONAL TIME : 0 mins
TOTAL TIME : 1 hour
YIELD : 28 servings

APPLE NUT WEDGES

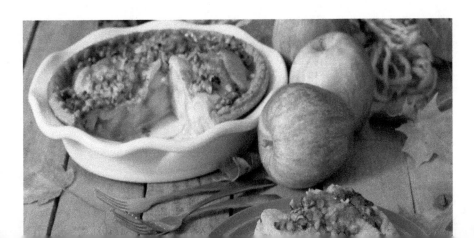

Apple Nut Wedges can be served warm with a dollop of a yogurt blend topping.

You can use MacIntosh apples for softer apple chunks. It's easy to prepare, diabetic-friendly, and it's super-duper delicious!

Enjoy!

- 1/8 teaspoon of salt
- 2 large apples, cored and chopped (2 cups)
- 1/2 cup of chopped walnuts or pecans, toasted
- 1/2 cup of light sour cream
- 1/4 cup of vanilla low-fat yogurt sweetened with artificial sweetener
- 1/2 teaspoon of vanilla
- Nonstick cooking spray
- 1 egg
- 2 egg whites
- 2/3 cup of packed brown sugar or brown sugar substitute blend equivalent to 2/3 cup of brown sugar
- 1 teaspoon of vanilla
- 1/3 cup of all-purpose flour
- 3/4 teaspoon of baking soda

PREPARATIONS

- Preheat oven to 325 degrees F.
- Use cooking spray to coat a 9-inch pie plate and set it aside.
- Combine egg whites, egg, brown sugar, and 1 teaspoon of vanilla in a large bowl.
- Beat with an electric mixer on medium speed until smooth, or for about 1 minute.
- Stir together baking soda, flour, and salt in a small bowl.
- Add flour mixture into the egg mixture. Stir until well combined.
- Fold in nuts and apples and spread batter evenly in the prepared pie plate.
- Bake until center is set, or for about 25 to 30 minutes.
- Slightly cool on a wire rack.
- For topping: whisk together yogurt, sour cream and 1/2 teaspoon of vanilla in a small bowl.
- To serve, cut dessert into wedges.
- Serve warm and enjoy.

PREP TIME : 25 mins
ADDITIONAL TIME : 0 mins
TOTAL TIME : 50 mins
YIELD : 8 servings

COCOA FUDGE COOKIES

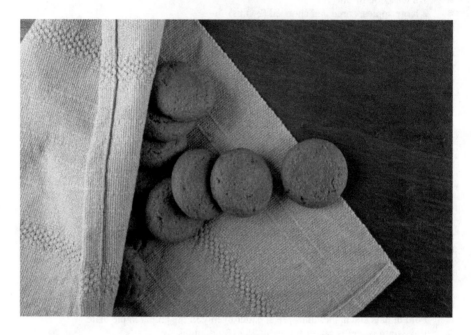

Cocoa Fudge Cookies is a dessert you can prepare in the saucepan. They are incredibly easy and freshly baked as well.

These cookies have crisp edges and chewy centers - so yummy.

You can make them with natural unsweetened cocoa powder or Dutch processed. I hope you love it, it would be great if you could give me feedback on them when you prepare it.

EASY DIABETIC DESSERT RECIPES

- 7 tablespoons of unsweetened cocoa
- 2/3 cup of granulated sugar
- 1/3 cup of packed brown sugar
- 1/3 cup of plain low-fat yogurt
- 1 cup of all-purpose flour
- 1/4 teaspoon of baking soda
- 1/8 teaspoon of salt
- 5 tablespoons of butter
- 1 teaspoon of vanilla extract cooking spray

PREPARATIONS

- Preheat oven to 350 degrees F.
- Spoon flour into a dry measuring cup.
- Level using a knife.
- Combine soda, flour, and salt; set it aside.
- In a large saucepan, melt butter over a medium heat.
- Remove from the heat; stir in sugars and cocoa powder.
- Add vanilla and yogurt, stir to combine.
- Add flour mixture, stir until moist.
- Drop level tablespoons 2 inches apart onto baking sheets coat with cooking spray.
- Bake at 350 degrees until almost set, or for about 8 to 10 minutes.
- Cool on pans until firm, or for about 2 to 3 minutes.
- Remove cookies from pans, cool on wire racks.
- Serve and enjoy.

PREP TIME : 20 mins
ADDITIONAL TIME : 0 mins
TOTAL TIME : 40 mins
YIELD : 2 dozen

THUMBPRINT COOKIES WITH RASPBERRY

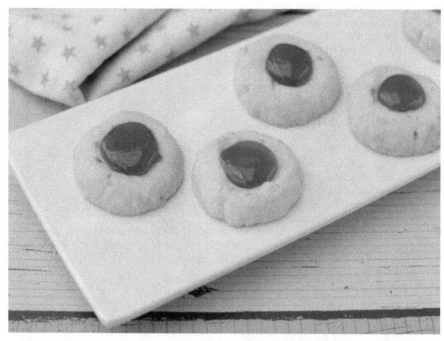

Adding some colors to your cookie tray with these jam-filled thumbprints will be so amazing. This recipe could be your healthy alternative for the next holiday, church gathering, or school party.

To save time, you can use pre-made raspberry jam to save time and they would be a hit. You need to add this to your favorites.

I hope you love it. Enjoy!

- 5 tablespoons butter, softened 1/4 teaspoon vanilla extract
- 1 large egg white
- 3/4 cup (3 ounces) grated almond paste 2/3 cup sugar
- 1 1/4 cups all-purpose flour (about 5 1/2 ounces) 1/4 teaspoon salt
- 6 tablespoons Raspberry Refrigerator Jam

PREPARATIONS

- Preheat the oven to 325 degrees F.
- Use parchment paper to line 2 large baking sheets, secure to baking sheet with masking top.
- In a bowl, place almond pasta, sugar and butter in a bowl.
- Beat with mixture at a medium speed until light and fluffy, or for about 4 minutes.
- Spoon flour into dry measuring cups and level using your knife.
- Add salt and flour until well combined and until golden.
- Remove cakes from the pans and cool on wire racks.
- Spoon about 1/2 teaspoon raspberry refrigerator jam in the center of each of the cookie.

Notes:
- Almond paste makes the dough pliable and moist.
- Look for it in the supermarket baking aisle.
- The large holes of box grater work well for grating the almond paste.
- To make deeper indentations in the cookies, use a wine cork.
- Bake both pans of the cookies at the same time.
- Rotate the pans in the oven halfway through baking time for even browning.
- Serve and enjoy.

PREP TIME : 20 mins
ADDITIONAL TIME : 0 mins
TOTAL TIME : 40 mins
YIELD : 2 dozen

SUGAR FREE BUCKEYE BALLS

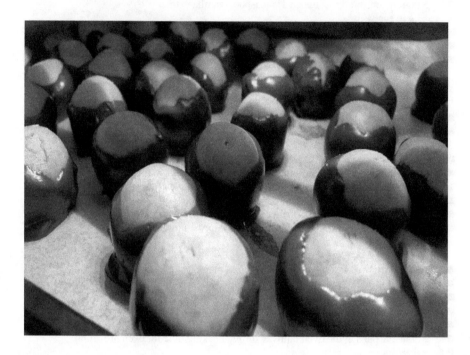

These delicious tasting Sugar Free Buckeye Balls are the perfect treat to share with your families and friends. They are low in carbs and diabetic-friendly because they're made with zero sugar.

We'll be adding sugar free peanut butter to this recipe. They actually work together in creating delicious taste.

INGREDIENTS

- 6 cups of Sugar Free Powdered Sugar
- 1 teaspoon of Vanilla Extract
- 1 1/2 cups of Sugar Free Peanut Butter
- 1 cup of Butter very soft
- 4 cups of Sugar Free Chocolate Chips

PREPARATIONS

- Prepare a baking sheet with wax paper. Set it aside.
- Cream together the sugar-free peanut butter, vanilla extract and sugar free powdered sugar in a mixing bowl.
- Form the mixture into 1 - 1 1/2-inches balls by rolling the dough in your hands.
- Place each of the ball on the wax prepared baking sheet.
- Place the prepared balls into the freezer for about 25 minutes, or until hard.
- Melt the chocolate in a microwave when you're ready to dip the balls in the chocolate or use the double boiler method.
- Stir the chocolate melts in well.
- Remove the peanut butter balls from the freezer and dip each of them into the chocolate. You can leave the area around where you can put your toothpick.
- Then place each ball back to the wax paper and refrigerate them.
- Melt more if you run low on chocolate.
- Serve and enjoy.

NOTE:
The buckeye balls should be stored in an airtight container in the refrigerator to keep them nice and fresh. Stored in this way they will keep for about 1 month. You can also freeze buckeyes in an airtight container or freezer Ziploc bag for up to 3 months.

PREP TIME : 20 mins
FREEZING TIME : 35 mins
TOTAL TIME : 55 mins
YIELD : 36 balls

BAKED APPLE CRISP

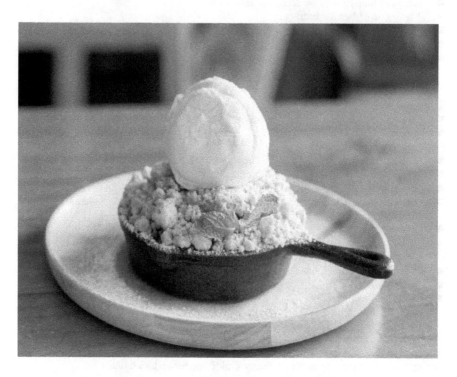

Are you wondering if you can bake this dessert on your grill?

Yes, you can. This is a traditional apple crisp that is baked directly on the grill. When you taste this recipe for the first time, you will be moved to add it to your favorite. It's so fantastic and a great addition to your Thanksgiving dinner.

It's yummy!

INGREDIENTS

- 2 teaspoons of ground cinnamon
- 2 teaspoons of baking powder
- 3/4 teaspoon of salt
- 1/2 cup (4 ounces) of butter
- 10 apples (about 5 pounds), preferably a mixture of Granny Smith and Golden Delicious
- 2 cups of all-purpose flour
- 1 cup of sugar
- 2 large eggs
- Vanilla ice cream (optional)

PREPARATIONS

- Melt butter over a low heat and set it aside.
- Peel, core and cut apples into 1/3-inch-thick slices.
- In a 9 by 13-inch baking pan, place apples and spread to be level.
- Mix flour, cinnamon, sugar, salt and baking powder in a bowl.
- Drop in eggs and mix with a fork or pastry blender until crumbly.
- Spread toppings evenly over apples.
- Drizzle with the melted butter.
- Prepare your grill for indirect heat at 350 degrees to 400 degrees F.
- On the grill, place the apple crisp and cover with barbecue.
- Cook until the apples are bubbling and the topping is browned, or for about 40 to 45 minutes.
- Serve warm with vanilla ice cream as an optional extra.
- **Apple Crisp:** Smoke this apple crisp if you really love the flavor of smoke.
- Cover 1/3 cup of apple-wood chips with water, then soak for 30 minutes and drain.
- Scatter the chips over the coals just before you place the apple crisp on the grate.
- Serve and enjoy.

PREP TIME : 10 mins
COOK TIME : 65 mins
TOTAL TIME : 85 mins
YIELD : 8 to 10 servings

CHEESE PITTAS

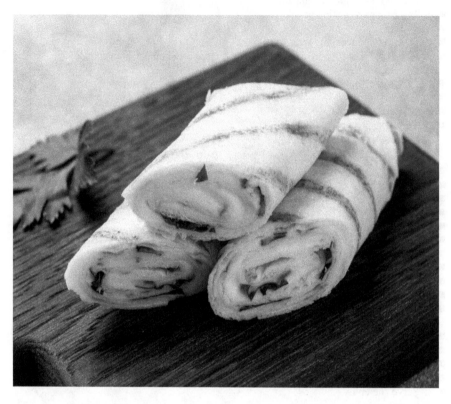

Cheese Pittas is one of my favorites. You can dump them into your favorite soup or have them together on their own for an easy and quick lunch that's always a hit.

With just six ingredients, your grilled cheese pitas can be ready-to-eat.

Cheese Pittas benefit from the absorbing, compressing, union-promoting nature of the astringent taste.

INGREDIENTS

- 1-2 teaspoon of butter or as needed
- 2 fluffy pittas or naan flat bread
- 4 slices of ripe tomato
- 2 handfuls baby spinach
- 4 ounces of grated cheese (you can use mozzarella with Havarti)
- salt and pepper to taste

PREPARATIONS

- Prep your cheese and veggies so they are ready to go.
- Heat a pan to medium high heat.
- Add 1 teaspoon of butter.
- Add a pitta to the pan once the butter begins to bubble.
- Top with spinach, cheese and tomato with a little extra cheese on the top.
- Top with the remaining pitta round.
- Now, grill.
- For an extra melty and hot center, pop a clear pot lid on top.
- Add another teaspoon of butter to the pan before flipping or you can feel free to spread it on top of the dry side of the pitta.
- If you're using one, pop your lid back and grill each side, or until it turns golden brown with a melty center.
- Cut into 4 wedges.
- Serve and enjoy.

PREP TIME : 5 mins
COOK TIME : 8 mins
TOTAL TIME : 13 mins
YIELD : 2 servings

FRUIT KABOBS

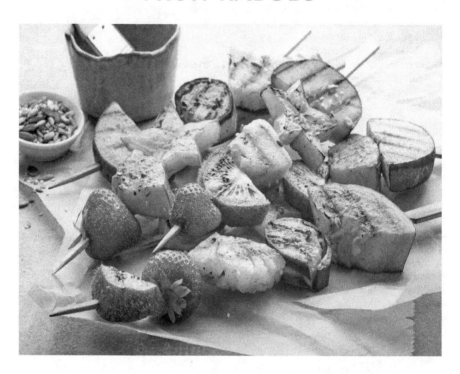

Do you know that grilling fruit caramelizes the natural sugars in them for a comfortable, sweet, and healthy dessert? It would be great if you try this grilled fruit kabobs this summer.

The natural sugars in the fruit will caramelize over the heat and bring out the fruit's sweet flavor. You'll realize that this recipe is a healthy and delicious dessert that tastes great. It not only just takes a couple of minutes on the grill, but it's so easy to prepare.

Serve it with a scoop of ice cream or some yogurt. You would love it!

- 1 cup of cantaloupe chunks cut into 1-inch pieces
- 1 cup of strawberries stems removed
- 1 cup of pineapple chunks cut into 1-inch pieces
- 1 banana cut 1-inch pieces
- Coconut oil spray
- 1 tablespoon of maple syrup for drizzling
- Vanilla yogurt for dipping (optional)

PREPARATIONS

- Inside water, soak the skewers for about 20 minutes to prevent the skewers from burning while grilling them.

Making the fruit kabobs:
- Thread 2 pieces each of pineapple, banana, cantaloupe and strawberry onto a skewer.
- Repeat this process to assemble as many skewers as you'd like to prepare.
- Drizzle with maple syrup and olive oil.
- Grill on a preheated grill until the fruit chars and softens, turning occasionally for about 10 minutes.
- Enjoy immediately.
- Dip in yogurt as an optional extra.

PREP TIME : 10 mins
COOK TIME : 2 mins
TOTAL TIME : 12 mins
YIELD : 6 servings

If you enjoyed this book, please let me know your thoughts by leaving a short review on **Amazon**

THANK YOU.

5 Easy Diabetic Dessert Recipes

Stella - Waters

CPSIA information can be obtained
at www.ICGtesting.com
Printed in the USA
LVHW051054210221
679518LV00003B/190